D1375754

ONE WEEK LOAN

Fourth Edition

First published 1989
Revised 2nd Edition 1992
Revised 3rd Edition 1995
Revised 4th Edition 1999

© Plane View Services Ltd, 22 Westview Grove, Wellington, New Zealand

ISBN 0-473-05765-4

Printing and typesetting: Hutcheson Bowman & Stewart Ltd

*To my wife Dawn
who encouraged me
to rewrite this book.*

THE AUTHOR

Brian R Mulligan qualified as a registered physiotherapist in 1954 and gained his Diploma of Manipulative Therapy in 1974. In 1996 he was made an Honorary Fellow of The New Zealand Society of Physiotherapists for his contribution to physiotherapy. In 1998 he was made a life member of The New Zealand College of Physiotherapy.

He together with R A McKenzie and J C Cameron established The New Zealand Manipulative Therapists' Association (now The New Zealand Manipulative Physiotherapists Association) in 1968 and was made a life member of this body in 1988.

Apart from his private practice in Wellington he has been involved in the teaching of manual therapy in New Zealand since 1970. He has been teaching Manual therapy internationally since 1972 and his courses have always proved popular. To meet the huge demand from therapists wishing to learn his techniques and to ensure high standards he set up an international organisation in 1995 to accredit teachers. It is titled 'The Mulligan Concept Teachers Association'. Participants on courses conducted by those accredited would be assured of a high and accurate teaching standard.

Brian Mulligan has been the author of numerous articles that have appeared in issues of the New Zealand Journal of Physiotherapy and overseas publications. Three videos are currently available.

'Mobilisations with Movement' was produced in 1993, it runs for over two hours and deals mainly with the extremity joints. 'Spinal Techniques, The Lumbar Spine and Thoracic Spine' and 'Spinal Techniques, The Cervical Spine' are two 90 minute videos produced in 1997.

CONTENTS

PREFACE

My book was first published in 1989. It was revised in 1992 and again in 1995. I make no apology for again revising it in 1999. There was new material to add and some old material to correct. In the new field of 'Mobilisation with Movement' we now have to include the rib cage and sacro-iliac joints. I have found in recent years that this new approach has been able to restore functional movements (in one treatment session) in joints after many years of restriction which questions the text books that speak of adaptive shortening.

Articles relating to the contents of this book are now appearing in our professional journals and I am particularly indebted to the authors of the scientific studies done on 'Tennis Elbow' (Vicenzino & Wright 1995) and Lateral Ankle Sprains (O'Brien & Vicenzino 1998).

The potential that exists in the new field of mobilisation with movement is enormous and more applications will evolve. As I stated in the last edition it began with "SNAGS" in the cervical spine which were in fact a mobilisation with active movement and from the cervical spine the techniques were later found to have a place in the treatment of certain thoracic and lumbar lesions. Extremity applications followed and as stated above, the rib cage and sacro-iliac joints are now with us. This revised edition will bring therapists up to date with the latest techniques using 'Mobilisations with Movement' (MWMS). The first part of the book deals with the spine, sacro-iliac joints and the rib cage and the second part deals with procedures for musculoskeletal conditions in other than the spine.

In writing a manual of this nature I am assuming that the reader . . .

a. Is fully acquainted with the contraindications to manual therapy and abides by the rules.
b. Has a sound knowledge of anatomy and biomechanics.
c. Complies with that special guideline "If you take up the slack in a joint before mobilising or manipulating and it is painful, do not proceed".
d. Has confident handling and language skills as without them the patient will not relax or comply with instructions. Poor handling can negate the advantages of manual therapy.

It is stating the obvious to say that many different manual therapy concepts and procedures are taught and all have a place in the treatment of patients.

However all the techniques in this publication, when indicated and used, are expected to bring about an immediate improvement in the patient's condition. If this does not occur I would suggest that the techniques are not appropriate for this patient or perhaps have not been undertaken correctly. On all of my courses I say to participants that if no improvement is evident at the time of delivery then discard the technique and try another approach. You should not continue to use them if some of the improvement gained is not retained between visits. Endless perseverance with no lasting benefit to the patient cannot be justified. Spectacular results are often obtained using MWMS and in my practice I expect at least one 'miracle' a day using these techniques.

REFERENCES

Bourdillon J F, Spinal Manipulation. London:William Heinemann Medical Books Ltd, 1970

Grieve G P, Modern Manual Therapy: Edinburgh, Churchill Livingstone, 1986

Kaltenborn F M, Mobilisation of the Extremity Joints. Oslo: Olaf Norlis Bokhandel, 1980

McConnell J, The Management of Chondromalacia Patellae-A Long Term Solution: Published proceedings of MTAA biennial conference Brisbane1985

McKenzie R A, The Lumbar Spine: Waikanae, Spinal Publications, 1981

Maitland G D, The Hypothesis of Adding Compression When Examining and Treating Synovial Joints: The Journal of Orthopaedic and Sports Physical Therapy: 2.1.1980

Mennell J McM, Joint Pain: Boston, Little Brown,1964

Mooney V, Where is the Pain Coming From?: Spine 12;8,1987

Mulligan B R, The Acute Wry Neck: New Zealand Journal of Physiotherapy. May, 1957

Mulligan B R, Plantar Fasciitis?: A Study Report: New Zealand Journal of Physiotherapy, November, 1973

Mulligan B R, The Painful Stiff Shoulder: New Zealand Journal of Physiotherapy, 4.7.1974

Mulligan B R, "SNAGS", Published papers IFOMT Congress, 1988

O'Brien T, *Vicenzino* B 1998 A study of the effects of Mulligan's Mobilization with Movement treatment of lateral ankle pain using a case study design. Manual Therapy 3(2):78-84

Vicenzino B, *Wright* A 1995 Effects of a novel manipulative therapy technique on tennis elbow : A single case study. Manual Therapy 1 : 30-35

PART ONE

I. SPINAL MOBILISATIONS

Introduction

It is interesting to note that in the field of manual therapy, when spinal manipulations are taught, attention is paid to the movement planes of the facet joints.

The direction of one's thrust is related to these planes especially when rotation and side flexion techniques are used. When one considers the various mobilisations that are taught much less attention is paid to the facet planes. These comments are generalisations, I know, but they lead me to say that the mobilisations that I use are always applied at right angles or parallel to the treatment planes of the facet joints. This complies with the rule that applies for extremity joint mobilisations as described in Freddy M Kaltenborn's book "Mobilisations of the Extremity Joints". Here he describes the treatment plane as lying across the concave articular surface.

The treatment plane moves with the concave partner. It behoves physiotherapists to be familiar with the direction of all spinal facet planes.

As you read further you will observe that my cervical and upper thoracic spinal mobilisations and nearly all spinal mobilisations with movement are done with the patient weight bearing. (In standing or sitting). I consider this to be extremely important as so often with non weight bearing techniques, improvements gained are lost when the patient resumes an erect posture. Although not covered in this text other forms of appropriate physiotherapy would be given concurrently by the author. At this juncture I must point out that I do not use my mobilisations on two regularly seen spinal conditions because there are more appropriate treatments available. These are the lumbar lesion producing a sciatic scoliosis (lateral shift) which is adequately dealt with using the R.A. McKenzie methods described in his book "The Lumbar Spine" and the acute wry neck (acute torticollis) which I will deal with separately.

A. THE CERVICAL AND UPPER THORACIC SPINES.

1. "NAGS"

Explanation

"NAGS" is the name I have given to oscillatory mobilisations which can be applied to the facet joints between Cervical 2 and Thoracic 3. It has become an acronym for Natural Apophyseal Glides. Although no problems will be encountered in the their execution in the cervical spine, therapists with short arms and small hands may not be able to use them in the upper thoracic spine.

"NAGS" are mid to end-range facet joint mobilisations that are applied antero-cranially along the treatment planes of the joints selected. They are graded according to the tolerance of the patient. They must never cause pain, maybe very slight discomfort. The patient is always seated which is a most convenient starting position. This is much more acceptable than prone lying especially with kyphotic patients. They can be combined with a little manual traction to render them more comfortable. They are used to increase spinal movement and decrease the pain associated with it. They are very useful in the elderly when applied with tender loving care. For the patient with grossly restricted cervical movement, they are a godsend, assuming that the loss of movement is not due to serious structural injury or other contraindicated pathology. They are also a good test for irritability. If a technique so subtle and gentle cannot be undertaken without pain then beware! To me this would mean that other forms of manual therapy would be contraindicated. Soreness after a manipulative procedure will usually be relieved by "NAGS". They are often used in conjunction with "SNAGS" or combined with "REVERSE NAGS" both of which will be described later.

Description (See figure 1)

The patient is seated comfortably on a stool or chair. To accommodate different sizes of patients it would help if the seat was height adjustable.

You, the therapist, (if right handed) stand at the right side of the patient so that your lower trunk is in contact with the antero-lateral surface of the patient's right shoulder. This is to stabilise the trunk of the patient when the mobilisation is carried out.

The patient's head is cradled against your upper abdomen and chest, comfortably held there with the right forearm diagonally positioned across the patient's left temporo-mandibular joint. In positioning the head, rotation and side flexion should be avoided. As the patient's head makes some contact with the lower chest, I always suggest that a female therapist may wish to place a soft pad between her chest and the patient's head. I always place a paper tissue between my white coat and the patient's face, not only for hygienic reasons, but to capture the cosmetics worn by some.

The middle phalanx of your right little finger is now placed (hooked) around the spinous process of the vertebra on top of the joint to be mobilised.(To mobilise the Cervical 5/6 joint your phalanx would be under the spinous process of Cervical 5).The right index, third and fourth fingers wrap around the occiput, if your hand is large enough, to maximise firm contact with the patient's head. With your feet apart, stand with most of your weight on your right leg. This, when the head is securely held, will apply a gentle and useful distraction to the cervical spine. The right arm also controls the degree of neck flexion. When some neck flexion is applied better contact can be made with the chosen spinous process. Remember that this alters the direction of the facet planes. It is almost impossible to make satisfactory contact with the spinous process of Cx 5 in a neutral position due to its proximity to the longer spinous process of Cx 6.

The lateral border of the thenar eminence of your left hand is now placed more under than over the little finger of your right hand. The required glide along the treatment plane can now be given, via your attached little finger, by pushing up and forward with your left hand towards the eyeball. Ensure that your little finger is relaxed, so that it only is being moved by your other hand, during the mobilisation. The patient's skull should remain perfectly still. The wrist of the left arm should be in extension with the forearm sloping in the direction of the facet planes. The glides are rhythmical (say three per second) and are undertaken through a mid to end range. Remember that the patient's trunk is stabilised by your body. Care must be taken to ensure that the glides follow the true direction of the treatment planes as failure to do so will produce pain. If one thrusts ventrally first before gliding up correctly in a cranio-ventral direction patients will experience unacceptable pain.

The mobilisations are repeated <6 times and then movements are reassessed. Sometimes several sets are required to bring about a change. As with all forms of manual therapy, if no improvement is discernible then some other form of therapy should be given. Of course you may have chosen the wrong level and with some patients several levels may be involved.

Remember, if the patient experiences some discomfort with "NAGS" make sure that you have applied a little traction by transferring more weight to your right leg. This should solve the discomfort problem.

The main advantage of this technique, apart from its efficacy, is its adaptability. The little finger may be placed over the articular pillar on one side to perform an unilateral glide to restore side flexion or rotation.

"NAGS" have been described by my colleagues who have mastered them as extremely useful and I would try them on most of my patients with cervical and upper dorsal problems particularly on those with a gross loss of movement or the elderly. Only once in twenty five years has a patient of mine had an adverse reaction to "NAGS". When this occurred I used "REVERSE NAGS" (to be described in the next section) and the patient was better immediately. This reaction was really memorable. A 37 year old man presented with bilateral neck pain and a marked loss of movement in all directions. I applied gentle "NAGS" and the result was a further reduction in his range of movement. "REVERSE NAGS" were then used and his symptoms virtually disappeared. After a second visit two days later no further therapy was required as he had fully recovered.

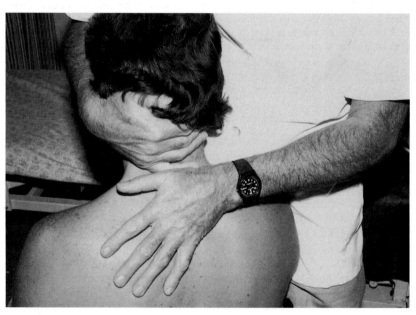

Figure 1
"NAGS" to the mid cervical spine.

2. "REVERSE NAGS"

Explanation

When teaching I claim that these mobilisations are the best in the world for the upper thoracic spine. They virtually replicate passively the head retraction exercises that we give to our patients with protruding heads. The patients describe them, when done properly, as 'great' and they feel their upper thoracic stiffness is being released.

As the name implies these mobilisations are the reverse of "NAGS". In the case of "NAGS" (say at Cx7/Th1) the superior facet glides up the inferior and with "REVERSE NAGS" the inferior facet glides up on the superior. If "NAGS" prove unsuccessful then this technique should be tried. It is useful in the lower cervical (Cx 6/7 down) but should be the treatment mobilisation of choice for the upper thoracic spine. I have never found them of value in the upper or middle cervical spines.

Description. (See figures 2a 2b and 2c)

The patient is seated. You stand beside patient and cradle his head to your body with the forearm. Place your fifth finger across the posterior part of the vertebra above the suspected lesion. The free hand's 3rd, 4th and 5th fingers are clenched. The I/P joints of the index are flexed and the MC/P joints of the thumb and index finger are extended. The thumb and index finger, spread in this way, will allow you to make contact with the prominent transverse processes on each side of an upper thoracic vertebra. You would proximate them to form a vee to make contact with the articular pillars of the lower cervical spine. A mobilisation takes place when you glide the inferior facet up on the superior one. This is achieved by thrusting up along the treatment plane with your bottom hand. For upper thoracic "REVERSE NAGS" you initially press firmly in to secure you thumb and index finger on the chosen segment's transverse processes and then glide cranially along the treatment plane. With "NAGS" the superior facet at the site of the lesion is moved up on the one below. With "REVERSE NAGS" the inferior facet moves up on the one above.

With a unilateral loss of end range neck rotation I would concentrate my "REVERSE NAGS" on the restricted side. It will prove successful with most patients.

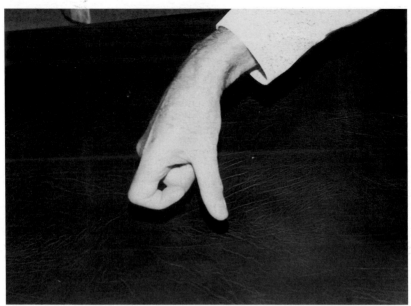

Figure 2a

The finger positioning for upper thoracic spine

Figure 2b

The finger positioning (vee) for lower cervical spine

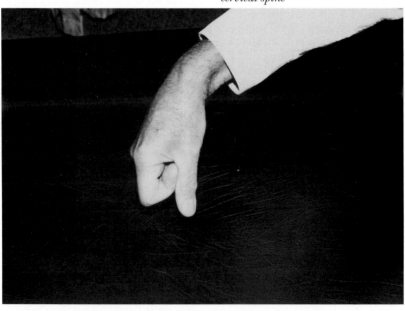

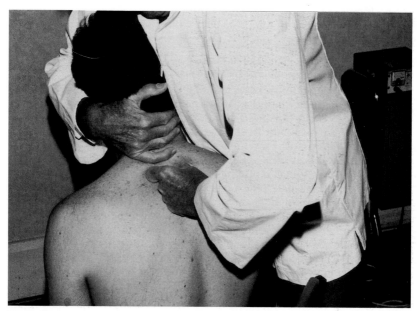

Figure 2c
"REVERSE NAGS" to the upper thoracic spine

3. "SNAGS"

Explanation

"SNAGS" is an acronym for "Sustained Natural Apophyseal Glides" and are useful as a treatment for the cervical and upper thoracic spines. "SNAGS" for the lumbar and thoracic spines will be described later. Cervical "SNAGS" were a learning experience for me. They were the first example of what has become a new approach in the field of manual therapy and that is the combination of mobilisations with movement (MWMS). What began as a unique technique for the cervical spine was found to have an important place in the treatment of other spinal joints, the rib cage and sacro-iliac joints . Because of their success there had to be a place for mobilisations with movement in the extremity joints and there certainly is. These will be dealt with under the extremity section of this book. "SNAGS" have yet to be scientifically vindicated but are never the less useful, safe, painless, easy to apply and a great introduction to this concept of mobilisation with movement. (The acronym has caught on. It is brief, explicit and when writing up case notes the only added description needed is to mention the level being treated. Thus my notes might say "SNAGS" right rotation Cx 6/7. If "SNAGS" were unilaterally applied this would be recorded thus; "SNAGS" left rotation (r) Cx 6/7.) To assist in the promotion of "SNAGS" and other mobilisations with movement I am gathering a library of video evidence of their usefulness as they are applied to patients in my clinic.

Although there are many wonderful texts available on spinal manual therapy I know of none that would meet all of the criteria that are detailed below and thus the claim they are a new approach.

1. They are weight bearing. All the texts that I have read on mobilisation have the patient lying. With "SNAGS" all procedures are done with the patient either sitting or standing. This has real advantages. When improvements take place in a functional posture they are more likely to be retained. Before using "SNAGS" I found that while more conventional mobilisations can result in an immediate improvement in function while the patient is lying, it is often lost when they resume a weightbearing posture.

2. They are mobilisations with active movement followed by passive over pressure. At the end of the attainable active range of movement, the patient must assist by applying overpressure with one of his free hands to further increase the movement. The over pressure is essential to gain the maximum benefit.

3. They follow the treatment plane rule. This rule must be observed. Trying to glide facet joints outside this plane is incorrect. You will find that patients will be unable to move their necks actively without pain if an incorrect glide is applied.

4. The mobilisation component is sustained. Most physiotherapy mobilisations for the spine are oscillatory. i.e. Maitland. "SNAGS" are mobilisations where the facet glides taking place are sustained while active movement, then overpressure, is taking place and these glides are maintained until the joint returns to the starting position. As an example, if Cervical 5/6 was being "SNAGGED" for a loss of extension then the therapist must sustain the glide with the movement until the neck resumes its resting position. Failure to do so might result in a painful response although no damage would occur.

5. They can be applied to most spinal joints. Yes they have a place in treating all the joints between the occiput and the sacrum.

6. When indicated they are **painless**. The indication for "SNAGS" is based on this statement, which is in fact **the rule governing their application.** An explanation to the patient and his co-operation is essential for them to be successful. If there is any pain with a mobilisation with movement then STOP. You will never exacerbate a patient's condition if you follow this rule. Remember of course that the pain may be produced because you have not followed the treatment plane rule or you may be mobilising the wrong segment.

7. They are carried out at end range. Mobilisations are usually undertaken with joints in a resting position. "SNAGS" are always involved with the end range of joint movement. If normal end range is lost, it is expected when applying "SNAGS" that the movement loss will disappear or be dramatically reduced and that no pain will be felt. If the restriction does not alter then you would be wasting your time to proceed further. Try some other form of manual therapy. These techniques are so good that when indicated an improvement will be observed with the very first mobilisation with movement.

8. There is a straight forward procedure for each movement loss. When familiar with the techniques you will immediately know which one to apply when there is a painful movement loss.

9. No time is wasted. Within a couple of minutes you can decide if "SNAGS" have a place in your treatment regime. If testing shows a painful loss of neck extension and right side flexion then "SNAGS" for these losses would be tried. Provided you are on the right level the pain with movement should go and the range increase straight away. If there is any pain check the level and technique. If still painful "SNAGS" would not be indicated. This routine takes only a short time.

Before continuing on, might I again remind the reader that "SNAGS" like other manual therapies are only part of the treatment program for patients presenting with musculo-skeletal disorders.

Description

The best way to describe all "SNAGS" techniques is to relate them to their application and this is how they will be dealt with.

As with all therapies an explanation must be given to the patient before treatment is undertaken. The success of "SNAGS" and all other techniques dealt with in this book is totally dependant on the co-operation of the patient. To oblige they must be fully conversant with what you are doing and the most important feature to stress is that the technique of combining mobilisation with movement MUST BE PAINLESS.

Pain of course may be experienced for many reasons and these must be checked out. As already mentioned you may have chosen the wrong level or the direction of your glide may be incorrect. Another point is that your handling rather than the technique may be at fault. If tissues are tender to the touch of your fingers or hands a thin layer of plastic foam may be placed under them. Finally "SNAGS" are not a cure all for all spinal mechanical disorders and should never be used if they produce pain.

(1) To increase rotation and/or decrease the pain associated with it. (See figure 3)

The patient is seated and you stand behind him. The medial border of one thumb's distal phalanx is placed on the tip of the spinous process of the vertebra above the suspected site of the lesion. The thumb nail would slope at approximately 45', in the direction of the eyeball. Your other thumb reinforces this. This means that if the patient has a lesion at Cervical 5/6 your

Figure 3

"SNAGS" for cervical rotation.

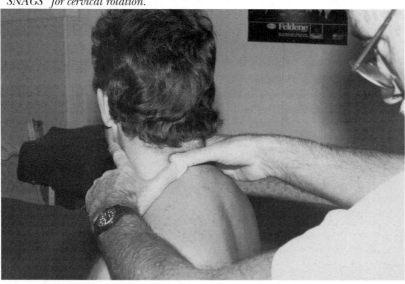

thumb would be on the Cervical 5's spinous process. The border of your thumb is used because the spinous processes are very small and the terminal pad would not be selective enough as it is too wide. Your other fingers are comfortably placed laterally on each side of the neck or upper antero-lateral thorax. You now glide the spinous process up in the direction of the treatment plane. (Towards the eyeball). The energy for this comes from the superimposed thumb pushing up on its partner. While this glide is being maintained ask the patient to turn his head slowly in the restricted painful direction. As the head rotates you must follow with your hands to ensure that the mobilisation with the movement taking place remains along the treatment plane. If "SNAGS" are indicated and the technique is correct the patient will be able to rotate his head further and feel no pain. Get the patient to apply overpressure. Sustain, for a few seconds, this new pain free end range of rotation, before returning to the midline. Repeat several times and then reassess. Unassisted active movement should now be much better.

"SNAGS" really are exciting when indicated. However do not over treat.

Once an improvement has been obtained on the patient's first visit, stop. As with other forms of manual therapy they are often sore the next day. However if this is the case the discomfort is of short duration and I would repeat the therapy two days later. Patients may complain of local tenderness under your thumb but if the right joint is being "SNAGGED" that is all that they will feel. It is rare for this technique not to assist but as with all forms of manual therapy if no change is apparent at the time of delivery then it should be abandoned. "SNAGS" are diagnostically helpful in inculpating the level(s) of involvement as pressure applied to the wrong level will make no difference. It is amazing that a weight bearing combination of active movement with mobilisation can be so demonstratively effective.

Variations

Since the first edition of this book was published we have found a very satisfactory way for patients to effectively "SELF SNAG" their cervical spines and this will be described later in this section.

When "SNAGS" are applied through the spinous process they are of course a bilateral technique. This is because both facets are equally glided. They can be effectively applied to the articular pillar on a chosen side. You still use your thumbs as you did over the spinous process. However when "SNAGGING" on the right, place your right thumb on the pillar and push up with your left. When "SNAGGING" on the left your left thumb would be on the pillar. Ensure that you get the direction right. It would seem more logical to apply them unilaterally as spinal lesions usually only involve one side. In the case of a patient with painful right rotation you would initially unilaterally "SNAG" on the right side. If this did not work then try the pillar on the left. If again you have no success then "SNAG" through the spinous process. Remember to further the efficacy of "SNAGS" for rotation have the patient apply overpressure by using one of his hands to push the head further round and sustain this position for a few seconds.

At this point in the text I would like to mention that there is a place for using "SNAGS" in the pain free, seemingly mobile, direction. (When you manipulate a cervical spine it is usually done in the pain free direction). The procedure is exactly the same as for rotation to the restricted and painful side but you do not have the feedback from the patient which ensures you are on the correct segment. What makes this variation really useful is overpressure at end range and this of course is done by the patient.

After say six "SNAGS" with overpressure there should be a marked improvement in neck function and if not use another technique.

(2). To increase side flexion and/or decrease the pain associated with this movement. (See figure 4)

The procedure is virtually the same as for rotation. The patient is seated. You stand behind the patient with your thumbs over the spinous process of the vertebra (as for rotation) above the suspected site. If Cx 5/6 then on Cervical 5. The patient slowly actively side flexes to the restricted and/or painful side, and just before the movement is felt to take place beneath the thumbs, you apply a sustained pressure up along the facet planes. It should not be painful. If it is you may not be on the correct level. With side flexion the vertebra tilts on the one beneath. You tilt your hands with it to ensure that as you push up, the upper facets move correctly.

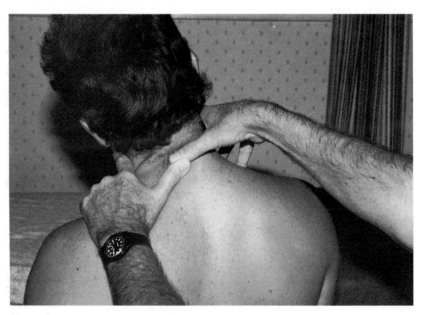

Figure 4

"SNAGS" for cervical side flexion. Patient can apply overpressure.

Variations

As with rotation the technique can be applied unilaterally on an articular pillar. This in fact, is now what we usually do as the patients can effectively "SELF SNAG" over the spinous process for side flexion. (Described later). Remember to have the patient apply side flexion overpressure with a hand pushing the head over and sustain this end range position for a few seconds.

(3). To increase extension and/or decrease the pain associated with it. (See Figure 5)

The procedure is almost identical to the two already described. The patient is seated and your thumbs are again used on the upper spinous process of the cervical segment involved. As the patient slowly extends his neck you push up along the facet treatment plane. Maintain this glide until the neck returns to the neutral position.

As will be repeated tediously over and over in this text no pain must be felt by the patient. If painful, "SNAGS" would not be used. Remember to try more than one level if your first choice is painful. There is a tendency to locate on the spinous process below the appropriate one or rather this has often be so in my case. However a repositioning of my thumbs has brought those exclamations of agreeable surprise from the patient.

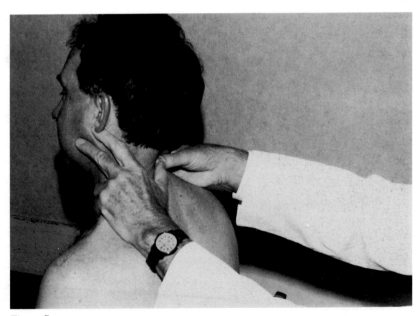

Figure 5

"SNAGS" for cervical extension (on the spinous process)

"SNAGS" for extension in the cervical spine will prove successful in more than 80% of patients. The technique is repeated six times and the movement reassessed. An important comment to make here is that when the neck moves into extension the facet joints now lie vertically. Allowances for this facet directional change must be made to ensure that you still glide up in the direction of the treatment plane.

Variation

As the neck moves into extension the spinous processes approximate making it difficult to stay effectively on the chosen site. This is especially true at the CX5/6 level or if you have a small neck to work with and your thumbs are of a generous size. This is when "SELF SNAGS" are marvellous. They are so good in fact that in my practice nearly all patients with extension problems are immediately taught to "SELF SNAG". (Dealt with later).

(4). To increase flexion and/or decrease the pain associated with this movement.

There are two techniques that can dramatically improve a loss of flexion. The first to be briefly described is, as you would expect, "SNAGS" but the second is quite different and is called "FIST TRACTION".

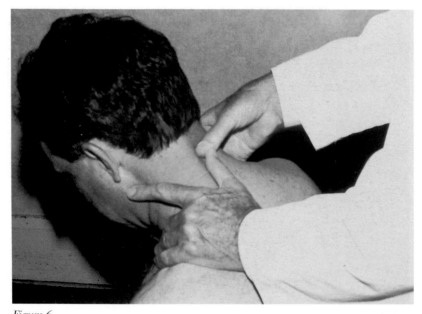

Figure 6

"SNAGS" for cervical flexion (on the spinous process)

"SNAGS" for flexion

You stand behind the seated patient with yes, one thumb reinforced by the other, placed over the superior spinous process of the spinal segment requiring therapy. As the patient flexes his neck you push up along the treatment plane. In full flexion the treatment plane will be nearly horizontal and this directional change must be remembered or your mobilisation will be ineffective and probably painful. Several repetitions should bring results. (See figure 6)

"FIST TRACTIONS" for flexion. (See figure 7)

These are ever so simple to do and in over 90% of patients who experience pain with mid to end range neck flexion you will find them successful.

The patient is seated. Now place your clenched fist under his chin in the following manner. The point of the chin rests on the circular plateau formed by your curled index finger and thumb. Your curled little finger is placed on the upper edge of the sternum. The patient is asked to place one hand around the base of his occiput and pull his head forward and down. The chin cannot

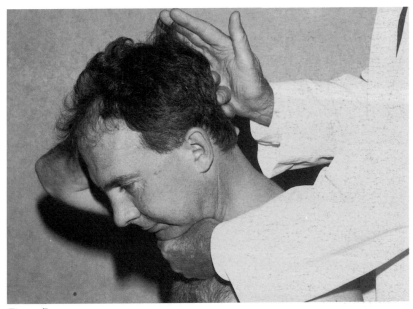

Figure 7
"FIST TRACTION" for cervical flexion.

move due to the wedging effect of your fist which becomes a fulcrum for a skull rotation resulting in a distraction of the facet joints in the lower cervical spine. He would maintain this traction effect for ten seconds and repeat three times. It must not hurt. If it did you would try something else. Your fist must be large enough to limit any painful flexion from taking place. If a fist is small or the neck being treated large then pain will be felt before the chin meets the fist and thus the therapy will not work. A useful tip in the case of a small hand is to place the palm of the free hand on the patient's sternum under the little finger effectively providing a better fulcrum. Another alternative is to place an appropriately thick book under the chin as a wedge. Patient's should be taught and encouraged to apply self "FIST TRACTION" as a home program. They can use their own fist while pulling the head forward with their free hand or use a book as a wedge. With the latter they can use both hands to apply the traction. They must always sustain the traction for at least ten seconds and repeat three times. "FIST TRACTIONS" are so good it is surprising that they were not thought of years ago.

If this technique does not work, and this is rare, the upper thoracic spine is probably where the problem lies. You would tend to suspect the upper thoracic spine if pain was only experienced with full neck flexion. A "SNAG" routine can be applied to this area. Stand behind the patient with your thumbs or the 5th meta-carpal, just distal to the pisaform, over the suspected thoracic vertebra's spinous process. As the patient flexes push up along the facet plane etc.

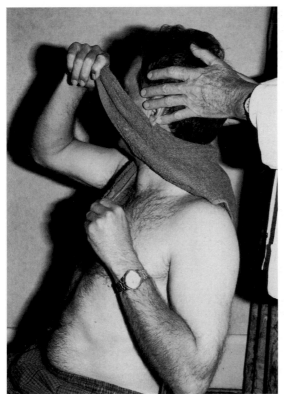

Figure 8
"SELF SNAGS" for cervical rotation.

4. "SELF SNAGS"

Explanation

Manual therapy, be it manipulation or mobilisation, is normally undertaken to restore function and most therapists ask their patients to follow up the treatment with an exercise routine. In the case of the cervical spine we have found "SELF SNAGS" very useful as a home routine. In fact they can be so successful that it is often the only manual technique used when a patient presents for treatment. It is a revenue reducing technique as it tends to speed up a patient's recovery. Before showing the patient how to "SELF SNAG" I explain on an articulated spine what the procedure is all about. They can see for themselves the structures clearly and understand the purpose of the exercise. "SELF SNAGS" can only be taught when the patient has his symptoms. Because of this I recommend that they be taught on day one before other measures are undertaken. This way the patient will get it right.

Descriptions

(1). "SELF SNAGS" for cervical rotation. (See Figure 8)

The only 'equipment' required is a small hand towel. The selvage on one side of the towel is hooked under the chosen spinous process. The ends of the towel on the same selvage side are now firmly held by the patient in the following manner. For right rotation grasp the left side of the towel with your right hand and the right side of the towel with your left hand. The left elbow is now hooked on the back of a chair to stabilise the arm and prevent thoracic rotation*. This is clearly seen in the photograph. The right hand now pulls the towel up in the direction of the facet planes (to eyeball) and the patient rotates his head to the right. When done properly the towel remains close to the side of the face. The upper right hand should position the towel so that it is close to the eye and keep it there as the movement takes place. As with "SNAGS" there must be no discomfort. If painful then try another level and check to ensure the direction of pull is accurate. To complete the therapy, rotation overpressure at end range must be applied by you the therapist or by someone in the patient's household. This assistance must not cause pain. After six to ten "SELF SNAGS" reassess and note the improvement. "SELF SNAGS" can be repeated two hourly initially if necessary. For left rotation the left hand would be on top to glide and pull the head around. We often get patients to "SELF SNAG" the incorrect level so that pain is felt with the active movement. They stop immediately and try other levels until they get it right.

Common mistakes that patients will make are...

(a) They forget to take their pulling hand around with the head when turning. This will give no relief from pain.

(b) They try to place the gathered towel over the spinous process instead of using the selvage. It is too bulky and not selective enough. When they pull up, one facet does not specifically slide up on its inferior partner. Another important point is that the pull must be on the selvage to ensure specificity.

(c) Another error is to pull the towel forward and not up in the direction of the facet plane.

(d) Finally they forget to maintain the glide until the neck returns from its journey to the right or left. If the pressure is removed before the return to the midline a sharp pain can be felt. This is undesirable.

As with "SNAGS", there is a place for "SELF SNAGS" in the seemingly mobile pain free direction. However to be really useful overpressure at end range is essential. This means that assistance would be needed from a spouse or friend.

* Hooking an elbow on the back of a chair was suggested by a New Zealand colleague (Zoe Clifford) and not mentioned in my earlier editions. There is no doubt that by doing this the technique is much better and I now teach it on all my courses.

(2). "SELF SNAGS" for side flexion or extension. (See Figure 9)

As for rotation the patient is seated and a small towel is used. The selvage on one side is hooked under the spinous process of Cervical 5 if the offending

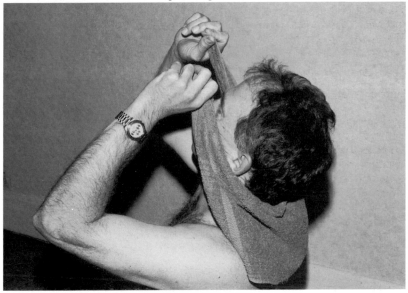

Figure 9

"SELF SNAGS" for cervical extension or side flexion.

segment is Cervical 5/6. The patient grips each end of the towel and pulls up along the treatment plane as he side flexes or extends his neck. When indicated the movement will increase and be pain free. It is repeated six to ten times and this routine could be undertaken every two hours or as you felt necessary. Pain and loss of extension is extremely common in patients presenting with cervical lesions. This "SELF SNAG" technique is so easy for the patient to do and so effective that in my practice it would be shown and used as a first step to improve extension instead of using "SNAGS". Remember to keep pulling the towel towards the eyeball as you extend, to maintain the facet glide along the treatment plane.

5. SPINAL MOBILISATIONS WITH ARM MOVEMENT.

("SMWAMS")

Introduction

I guess this had to happen. Mobilisations with movement (MWMS) began in the cervical spine when I developed "SNAGS" which of course are spinal mobilisations with spinal movements. From the spine I found they had an important role to play in the peripheral joints by combining extremity joint mobilisations with extremity joint movements. (You will read of these later in this book). What I have now found is that there is a place in manual therapy for combining a sustained spinal mobilisation with an extremity movement. In this section I will address their use in the upper extremity.

This new technique should be considered as a therapy when a patient presents with a pain that is experienced with an upper extremity movement that could be of spinal origin.

Examples could be :

1. Pain radiating from the upper fibres of trapezius to the forearm when the arm is abducted above the horizontal.

2. Rhomboid pain felt by the patient when the arm is adducted across the body in the horizontal plane.

3. Pain radiating down to the hand with arm movements that involve moving the shoulder girdle.

This new mobilisation with movement developed because of the fact that when the shoulder girdle is moved, spinal movement also takes place because of the muscle attachments from the scapula to the cervical and upper thoracic vertebrae. You can prove this while reading this book. Place an index finger on say the spinous process of Cervical 7 and then moving your free arm above the horizontal to involve the shoulder girdle. Agree?

This new technique is very simple to apply and should be used as part of your assessment as it has a diagnostic significance as well as being a therapy.

Description. (See figure 10a and 10b)

To describe the basic technique let us assume your patient has pain radiating down to the flexor area of the right forearm when he horizontally adducts his shoulder.

You stand behind the seated patient. Because of the pain distribution, (Cervical 5) initially place the medial border of your left thumb, on the right side of the spinous process of the 4th cervical vertebra. Place your right thumb on the other border on your thumb. Your outer thumb pushes on its partner to

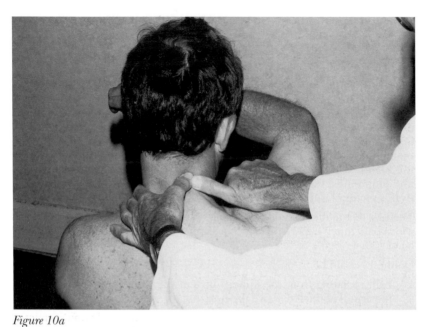

Figure 10a

"SMWAMS" In this case the spinous process of cervical 4 is moved to the left with right horizontal adduction.

Figure 10b

"SMWAMS" using index finger to push on thumb with arm abduction.

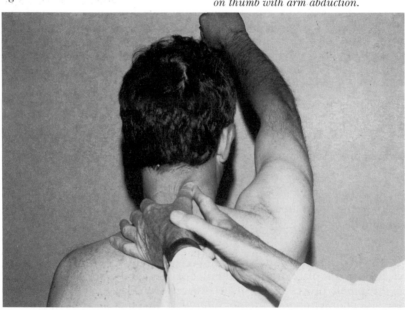

move the spinous process across to the left and sustain this rotation as the patient horizontally adducts his right arm.

You will see from the figure 10a that the thumb lies obliquely on the side of the neck as that is how the spinous process lies. Try to make as much contact with the spinous process as your thumb will allow and not just the bifid tip which will hurt. If you are on the correct vertebra and the technique is appropriate the patient will feel no pain at all. After several repetitions the patient should then be able to move his arm in the offending direction without symptoms and without the accompanying sustained mobilisation. If this were not so then the treatment would be discarded. When successful two more sets of these pain free spinal mobilisations with arm movement (SMWAMS) would be undertaken.

If the offending movement was abduction then I would reinforce the thumb on the spinous process, with my index finger. This way I can keep my hand off the top of the shoulder girdle and thus not be in the way of the fully abducting arm. (See figure 10b)

Remember if there is any pain when the arm is moved do not proceed. Instead try the spinous process above or below your first choice in case you have chosen the incorrect level. When the patient is moving his arm, it is necessary that enough momentum is used to ensure that a vertebral movement takes place at the segment you are trying to influence. Sensible patients can be taught to treat their own necks by placing a middle finger on the side of the vertebra and pulling it across , as you did, as they move the arm that is involved. (I place a small piece of tape on the neck to assist the patient find the level when they are doing the above as a home program). The technique replicates what you did with them. They would be instructed to repeat the therapy several times a day as you deem is necessary. Another point to make is that the patient must hold his head in a good postural position while being treated. There is a tendency for the patient to flex his neck when your thumb is positioned, which tightens the posterior structures and makes your therapy ineffectual.

This technique can be used on the upper thoracic spine when the patient's upper thoracic pain is provoked with arm movement.

As with all MWMS it must be stressed that the glide in the chosen direction must not be released until the patient's arm returns to the starting position. This rule is very important.

Rationale

When you move, say the spinous process of Cervical 4 to the right, Cervical 4 rotates to the left on Cervical 5. This causes the facets of Cervical 4/5 on the left to separate and reposition. Now, when the left arm is raised above shoulder level, the muscle attachments from the scapula to the spine will make the thoracic and cervical vertebrae move up to the level of Cervical 4 which you have rotated to the left. At the level of Cervical 4/5 a mobilisation/manipulation takes place that cannot be replicated by any other means. It causes an unique biomechanical effect which can prove extremely valuable therapeutically. Often an audible "click" can be heard similar to that which can be heard when you manipulate a facet joint.

Summary

These spinal mobilisations with arm movement are extremely effective when indicated, and thus really exciting and are completely safe if basic rules are followed. These are:

1. When indicated no pain is experienced with the technique.

2. After 6 to 10 repetitions of the arm movement with sustained spinal mobilisation the patient should notice a marked improvement in arm function. If not, try another therapy.

3. Do not over treat. The quick change for the better in the status of the patient's symptoms may inspire the therapist to over treat. On day one, if I have any concern about the patient, I may only use one set of SMWAMS and review the patient a couple of days later.

4. As already stated, do not release your mobilisation until the patient has returned to the starting position.

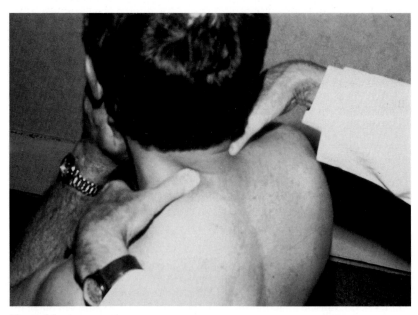

Figure 11

"MWM" at cervical 5/6 with right rotation. Note overpressure

6. OTHER MOBILISATIONS WITH MOVEMENT TECHNIQUES (MWMS) FOR THE CERVICAL AND UPPER THORACIC SPINES

Introduction

"SNAGS", as already described, are a mobilisation with movement but there is another MWM that I would use every day in my practice that is extremely useful. In fact it would be my first choice as a manual therapy on patients presenting with pain and stiffness of Cx 5/6 and Cx 6/7 origin. As you know the most common levels of cervical degeneration are at these segments. Computer users, the desk bound and those with protruding neck postures show up in high numbers with the above symptoms. Many are middle aged or older but there are an increasing number of younger patients requiring treatment because they spend hours at a computer. It goes without question that postural exercises and management plus a workstation review must be dealt with. Might I suggest, at this stage, you take an articulated spine and move the spinous process of Cx5 to the left and the spinous process of Cx6 to the right. You will observe that the Cx 5/6 facet joint on the right is separated. This is not a natural movement for the spine. It is while this repositioning of the segment is sustained that the patient is asked to move his neck.

Description

We will assume that the patient has a painful loss of right rotation and his discomfort is felt in the adjacent muscles and Cx 5/6 is the offending joint.

You stand behind the seated patient and place the end of your right thumb to the right of the spinous process of Cx 5 and your left thumb to the left of Cx 6 (See figure 11). In doing this, start with your thumbs on the articular pillars and gather up the posterior muscle bulk as you move to make contact with the spinous processes.

By moving your thumbs transversely across you effect a rotation to the right of Cx 5 on Cx 6. Concurrently you ask the patient to actively rotate to the right. As with all techniques the patient should experience no pain and to enhance the treatment have him give the necessary overpressure by pushing his head around. (If there was pain with the movement you may have chosen the wrong level).

After six repetitions there should be improved function to the satisfaction of both you and the patient. If no change? Yes, you would try another technique. Well done.

Handling. If the thumb pressure is uncomfortable have a small piece of plastic foam between the tips of your thumbs and the patient's skin.

In the section 5. SMWAMS were dealt with. Sometimes, when say moving Cx5 to the left proves ineffective with right arm movement, try moving the spinous process of Cx6 to the right at the same time as just described in this section. You may find the arm now moves painlessly. This is probably because just pushing on one spinous process was not enough to bring a useful positional change to allow the expected pain free arm movement.

B THE UPPER CERVICAL SPINE - SPECIAL THERAPIES

In this section I wish to deal with three specific conditions. They are "Acute Wry Neck", "Headaches" and "Vertigo".

1. THE ACUTE WRY NECK

In the May 1957 issue of the New Zealand Journal of Physiotherapy (3) I had an article published on this condition and since that time I have always used the method about to be described as it is always successful. We all know the condition is self limiting and will spontaneously recover within three or four days. The pain is unilateral, confined to the neck, is common in the young and is so distressing that patients usually seek medical attention. Because of the spasm encountered I consider manipulation unkind and unnecessary. The procedure I use is as follows.

The patient lies supine with his head on a pillow on which has been placed a hot pack or whatever. He rests for a minute or two and then begins exercising his head in rotation to the painful restricted side. The range of movement is encouraged by small slow oscillations up to the pain block. It is a small teasing motion at the end of the range. Although discomfort is experienced it should never be so strong a movement as to be considered painful. Within 5 minutes of exercising the spasm slowly starts to diminish and the range of movement increases. In every case within 20 minutes (or less) a full range of painless movement will have returned. The patient will still experience pain with side flexion. On standing the neck will still be painful but much better. He should rest that day and not return to work or school. We tell the patient that when he gets home to apply a folded pillow case collar. Before going to sleep that night I suggest they remove the collar, lie with the head on a pillow and repeat the exercise routine that they undertook in my clinic. The collar is then replaced for the night. The next morning they can expect to be 90% better. Rarely do we have to see a patient more than once. If this form of therapy did not work I would respectively suggest that the patient does not have an Acute Wry Neck.

Remember that a wry neck does not produce a headache, there are no radicular signs and the pain is unilateral.

2. HEADACHES
Explanation

The treatments for patients plagued by headaches has been of special interest to me for three decades. However I will confine comments on this subject to my special tests and treatments for this condition including a "SNAGS" technique that we find useful in restoring a loss of Cervical 1/2 (atlas/axis) rotation which is often associated with a headache.

If a patient is suffering from a headache of upper cervical origin then one of the mobilisations or the traction to be described should, as it is being applied, stop the pain. They are sustained techniques. I assume that if a headache stops with a manual technique involving the upper cervical spine then this must be diagnostically significant as to the site of the lesion causing the problem and the fact that there is a mechanical component.

The first technique is like the "NAGS" mobilisations already covered but differs in that the top two vertebrae are moved ventrally on the base of the stationary occiput above. The second is where the occiput is drawn forward on the upper cervical spine. The third is a form of manual traction which distracts the upper cervical facets at right angles to their treatment planes. The fourth as already mentioned is a mobilisation with movement that can restore a loss of Cervical 1/2 rotation.

Descriptions

(1). "HEADACHE SNAGS" . (See Figures 12 a and b)

You stand beside the seated patient. His head is cradled between your body and the right forearm if you stand on his right side. (See earlier description of head position for "NAGS"). The right index and middle and ring fingers wrap around the base of the occiput and the middle phalanx of the little finger lies over the spinous process of Cx 2. (It is prominent and is the first process palpable 2.5cms below the occiput). The lateral border of the left thenar eminence lies over the right little finger. Pressure is now applied in a ventral direction on the spinous process of Cervical 2 while the skull remains still due to the control of your right forearm. The really gentle moving force to do this comes from your left arm via the thenar eminence over the little finger on the spine of Cx 2. The first thing that happens is that the second vertebra moves forward on the first until the slack is taken up, then the first vertebra moves forward on the base of the skull. This is quietly taken forward until end range is felt and this position is maintained for at least ten seconds. If indicated the headache will lift and you have two ways now to deal with it. The first is for you to manually repeat the "HEADACHE SNAGS" six to ten times. The second is to have the patient "SELF HEADACHE SNAG" . This is achieved by placing the now familiar hand towel around the spinous process

---

Manual Therapy

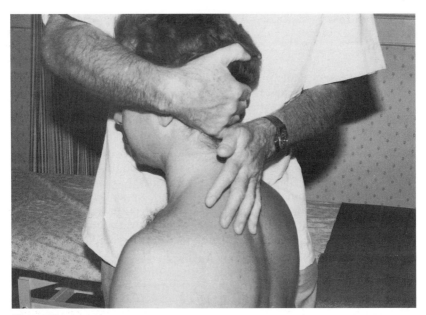

Figure 12a

"HEADACHE SNAGS"

Figure 12b

"SELF HEADACHE SNAGS"

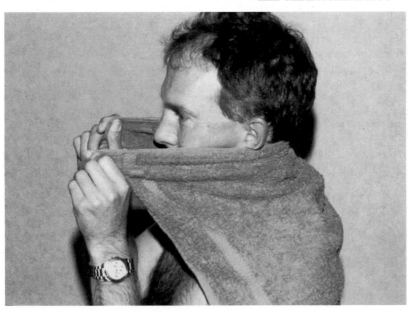

of Cervical 2 and securing it with the hands. The patient now glides his head back without tilting it which will replicate what you the therapist did with the "HEADACHE SNAG". This is not a strong procedure as excessive muscle activity between the occiput and the spine would be counterproductive. The patient sustains the posterior glide for at least ten seconds and repeats the process six to ten times. They should now feel much better. The technique can be repeated as often as you feel necessary during the day. Remember that the facet planes we are dealing with here lie in an antero-posterior direction and do not slope upwards like their lower relations.

Important. When applying the "Headache Snag" the good manual therapist will imperceptibly alter the direction of the glide to effect a change. Small adjustments in direction may be necessary as the true facet plane directions vary with individuals.

"Woolly head" sensation. If patients experience what they describe as a woolly sensation in the head, after an upper cervical manipulation, "HEADACHE SNAGS" should be used. They will often, after a few repetitions, rid the patients of their distress.

(2). "REVERSE HEADACHE SNAGS". (See Figure 13)

The patient is seated with the head held in the manner described previously, except that the right little finger is wrapped around the base of the occiput

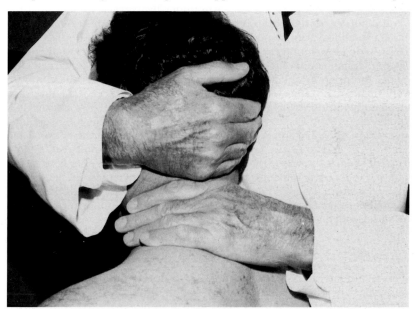

Figure 13
"REVERSE HEADACHE SNAGS"

and makes no contact with the cervical spine. The thumb and index finger of the left hand wraps around Cervical 2 so that the web between them is in contact with the posterior part of the neck. The spine is thus held securely. The grip should be comfortable and care taken not to "throttle" the patient. While the upper cervical spine is stabilised in this manner, the head is taken forward on the column to end range and held there for at least ten seconds. In moving the skull you must not tilt it to ensure that the facet planes remain parallel. If this technique is indicated the headache will go and several repeat mobilisations should be undertaken. As you will have noted this technique is the reverse of the previous one. A Sydney colleague suggested, when I was teaching there, that the same effect could perhaps be achieved by the patient, if he were to wrap a towel around his occiput to stabilise it, and then glide his neck posteriorly. I would agree. Self "FIST TRACTION" are often useful when patients respond to "REVERSE HEADACHE SNAGS".

(3). UPPER CERVICAL TRACTION (See Figures 14a and b)

For many headaches, that are the result of a biomechanical problem in the upper cervical spine, traction in slight extension is the treatment of choice. Remember when dealing with facet joints any traction being applied must take place at right angles to the treatment plane. The testing technique to be described complies with this rule when applying a distraction to the atlanto-occipital and atlas-axis joints. The patient lies supine and you place the lower section of your right (or left) forearm under his cervical spine so that the ventral border of your radius is tucked under the base of his occiput. If you have a small forearm, or perhaps the patient is large, you can place a narrowly folded towel under your arm to raise it a little. No place two fingers of your other hand under his chin. To apply traction pronate the forearm tucked under the occiput, while delivering an equal pressure under the chin with your fingers. The effect will be a distraction of the upper cervical joints while the natural lordosis is maintaned due to the positioning of the forearm. Hold the traction for at least ten seconds and see if the headache goes. Very little distraction is needed and care must be taken to ensure that the occipital and chin forces equate or the head will tilt and the desired effect will be lost. Experience has shown me that over 90% of headaches of upper cervical origin that I see, cease while this type of traction is being applied. On this basis alone it is worth trying. When effective it is easy to set up a sustained traction treatment using a cervical harness, a small weight and supporting the lordosis with a rolled up towel.

(4). "SNAGS" for restricted Cervical 1/2 rotation. (See Figure 15a)

This technique can be extremely useful in restoring upper cervical rotation and especially when manipulation is contraindicated or the therapist does not have manipulative skills. Most patients can be taught to "SELF SNAG" which is a bonus. These days a "SELF SNAGS" is my treatment of choice.

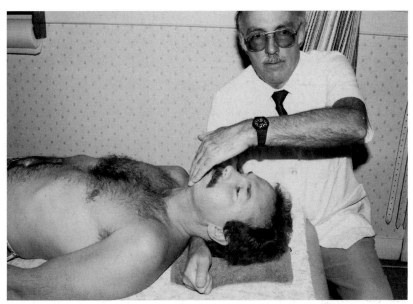

Figure 14a
Upper cervical traction. Test and treatment.

Figure 14b
Upper cervical traction in extension with harness. Note rolled towel.

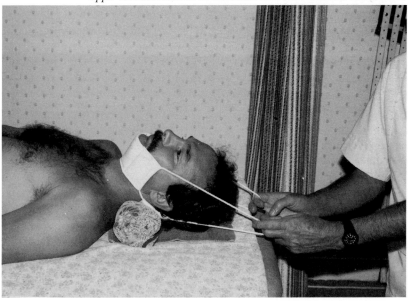

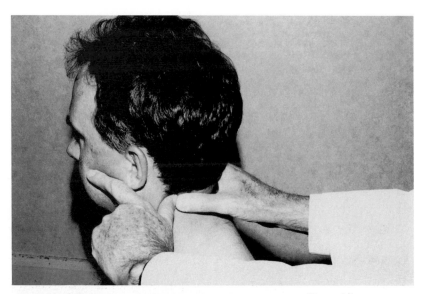

Figure 15a

"SNAGS" for restricted rotation at Cervical 1/ 2.

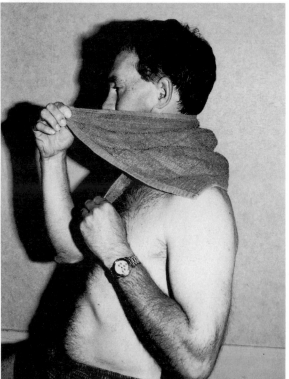

Figure 15b

"SELF SNAGS" for restricted rotation at Cervical 1/2.

Manual Therapy

The patient is seated and you stand behind him. Let us assume he has lost right Cervical 1/2 rotation. You place the pad of the terminal phalanx of your left thumb as far laterally as you can on the transverse process of Cervical 1 on the left. This is large and readily palpated just below the ear lobe. Your right thumb is now placed over your left. The patient is asked to slowly rotate his head to the right while you provide a gliding force ventrally on Cervical 1 with your thumbs to assist the movement. As the head rotates your thumbs must move around with it to remain on "target". There must be no pain as is the rule for all "SNAG" techniques. Remember that the treatment plane at this level is almost horizontal when the patient is seated. Thumb pressure is not released until the neck returns to the mid line. If this did not work then you would "SNAG" the Cx1 transverse process on the right with rotation to the right.

"**SELF SNAGS**" for Cervical 1/2 rotation. These are **brilliant**!

For these a small towel is required as was the case with the other cervical joints already dealt with. The selvage on one side is placed around the back of the neck immediately below the occiput so that it lies over Cervical 1. As a guideline, level with the tip of the ear lobe and top teeth. For right rotation the patient holds the end of the towel on the left with his right hand and the end of the towel on the right with his left hand. Hook the bent right elbow on the back of a chair. The right hand should be above the left. As the patient turns his head to the right his right hand assists Cervical 1 to rotate by pulling it round. (See Figure 15b). It must not hurt, cause nausea or giddiness. At this stage the patient gets his partner to apply overpressure to the movement. The over pressure should produce no discomfort. On day one, in my rooms, I would only do this twice and reassess. If it proves successful the patient can be instructed to repeat sets of six frequently during the day or as you think fit. If sore, reposition the towel to check if the placement of the towel was the problem. By repositioning I mean raise or lower it just a few millimetres.

(2). VERTIGO, NAUSEA AND OTHER "VERTEBRAL ARTERY" SIGNS

Explanation

Vertebral artery signs are a contraindication to manipulation and all manual therapists are aware of the protocols that exist to test for these signs. However there are simple mobilisations with movement that you can do which will often bring about a safe resolution to the patient's problem. This treatment is only applied when the vertigo or other signs are produced with neck movement and it is usually neck extension that most commonly causes giddiness. However rotation can also be a problem as can flexion. I have yet to see a patient that experiences vertigo etc. with both left and right rotation even though they may have symptoms with both flexion and extension movements.

Description

Before the treatment is tried you must ensure that you have the full co-operation of the patient. He will be asked to move his head in the direction that produces his symptoms, provided that with mobilisation this movement is symptom free. He STOPS the movement if it produces giddiness or other vertebral artery signs. As with all "SNAGS" techniques they are only used if they are symptom free. If you follow this rule you will never exacerbate a patient's condition.

If extension causes the problem.

Stand behind the seated patient. Place the palmar aspect of the first phalanx of one thumb reinforced by the other over the spinous process of Cervical 2. Your free fingers apply a slight pressure to the sides of the face to stabilise the skull as you now push ventrally on Cx2 and then have the patient slowly extend his neck. (See figure 16) Remember to tilt with them as the movement takes place. The patient should now be able to extend his neck, symptom free. The forward thumb pressure is sustained until the neck returns to the starting position. Repeat the mobilisation with movement six times. The patient should now be able to extend his neck without experiencing vertigo or nausea. That would be all you would do by way of manual therapy on day one.

An alternative way would be to make use of the "headache SNAG" procedure. Instead of very very gently gliding Cx 2 forward do so more firmly and then have the patient extend his neck provided he is symptom free.

(Perhaps in this text it should be mentioned that patients who have problems with their necks in bed should be supplied with a soft collar to sleep in. In my practice we advise patients to fold an empty pillow case in half lengthways and then into three so you have long narrow scarf. Wrap it around the neck securing it with a safety pin. It is amazing how effective the pillow case collar is).

If the patient is reasonably intelligent you must show him how to "SELF SNAG" his neck so that the treatment can be repeated several times a day should this be necessary. The procedure with the small towel is the same as for a loss of neck extension. However you keep the towel parallel with the upper jaw as you move into extension, because of the treatment plane. Some patients only require one treatment, others may require three or four but when this technique is indicated and used the patient always makes a rapid recovery.

If left rotation is the offending movement you have two thumb positional choices.

(1). Place your left thumb reinforced by the other, on the transverse process of Cervical 1 on the left side. It is easy to palpate just below the ear lobe. Before the patient rotates in the offending left direction you push the process forward with your thumbs, being mindful of the treatment plane. Now the patient turn his head to the left slowly provided no symptoms appear. If symptom free he applies overpressure. After one or two

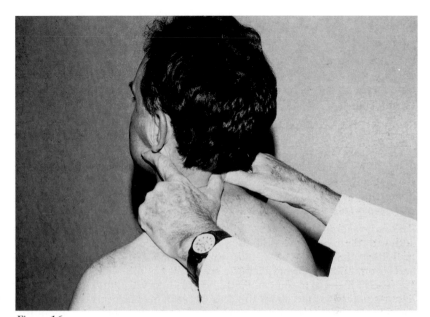

Figure 16

"SNAGS" for nausea or vertigo with extension

"SNAGS" he should feel much better. More "SNAGS" would be given on any subsequent treatment sessions should they be required.

(2). Repeat the left rotation with your thumbs on the right side.

I have found that when the patient has 'vertebral artery signs' with rotation, thumb placement on the offending side has been the most successful. The reader will note that we used the same "SNAG" technique to restore Cervical 1/2 rotation. (See figure 15a)

Remember that visual disturbances associated with neck movement can also respond to these techniques.

Physiotherapy really does get more satisfying as the years pass. Why do these techniques work? The explanation that I give to my patients is that their vertigo is due to a gliding malfunction in one or more of the joints in the upper cervical spine. The easiest way to demonstrate this is to use an articulated spine.

C. THE LUMBAR SPINE

1. "SNAGS"

Introduction

"SNAGS" in the treatment of the lumbar spine added a new dimension to my therapies for this area. They have proved so exciting to use when indicated and because of this some theorising became inevitable when wondering how a procedure can be so useful. However we all know that it is unwise to print one's theories because if they can be faulted the author's credibility is questioned and any valid treatment claims made could be cast aside. Anyway the reader may find my following comments of interest.

Different manual therapy schools of thought have thrived through the decades with their respective followers and this has bothered those of us with orthodox minds. We read of facet theories, disc theories, muscle theories and so on. Today gaining scientific acceptance is the McKenzie treatment approach which fits in so neatly with the disc theory. Up until now one thing has always puzzled me about the disc theory. This has been the fact that a simple facet manipulation can sometimes bring great relief to a patient that we 'know' has a minor disc lesion. I will now offer one hypothesis which I feel ties in facet hypomobility with disc involvement. It explains why "SNAGS", which I believe work directly on facet joints, can help a disc lesion and certainly assist with the response to a McKenzie or other routine. These remarks definitely pertain to the lumbar spine.

During normal flexion of the spine the disc distorts and becomes wedge shaped. The vertebral bodies proximate ventrally and separate dorsally. The nucleus (or whatever) moves posteriorly, but the disc whose volume is unalterable, remains under the umbrella of the vertebra above. (See figure 17). For this to occur the facets joints must be mobile. If the facet joints are hypomobile, when flexion takes place, the vertebral bodies will be able to proximate anteriorly but unable to separate dorsally. The disc may no longer remain under the umbrella of the vertebra above and instead bulge posteriorly causing symptoms. These symptoms would all be a matter of degree. If there was a weakness in the posterior wall of the disc then even greater problems would arise from facet hypomobility. What I am implying is that most back pain comes from the disc which is producing symptoms due in no small measure to the facets. When you have a patient, who has pain to the lateral lower leg with spinal flexion standing, and you "SNAG" him, and while doing so his leg pain disappears, you will probably support my hypothesis.

As with all techniques an explanation must be given to the patients. This is really important in the lumbar spine as a lack of understanding could lead to an exacerbation of their pain and without their co-operation the procedures will not work. You tell patients that you are going to move a vertebra with your hand in such a way that the pain they feel with a particular movement

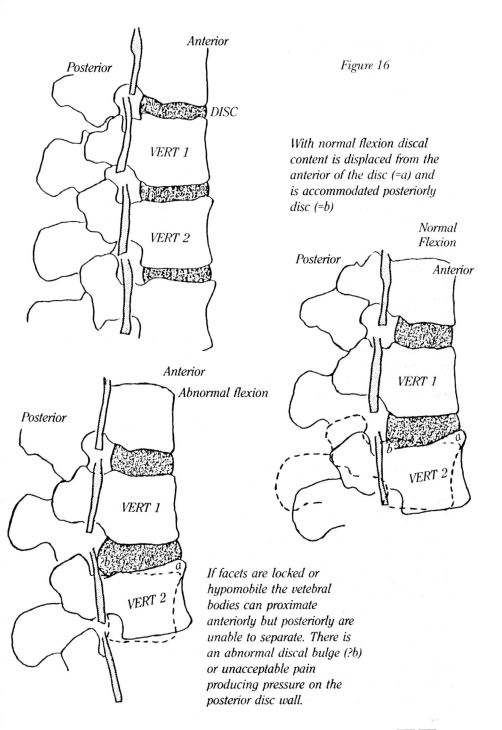

Anterior

Posterior

Figure 16

DISC

VERT 1

VERT 2

With normal flexion discal
content is displaced from the
anterior of the disc (=a) and
is accommodated posteriorly
disc (=b)

Normal
Flexion

Posterior

Anterior

VERT 1

b

a

VERT 2

Anterior

Abnormal flexion

Posterior

VERT 1

b

a

VERT 2

If facets are locked or
hypomobile the vetebral
bodies can proximate
anteriorly but posteriorly are
unable to separate. There is
an abnormal discal bulge (?b)
or unacceptable pain
producing pressure on the
posterior disc wall.

will disappear. If they feel any pain they must tell you so that you can check your technique or try another level. Without their help "SNAGS" are valueless. I must say at this point, do not overdo the "SNAGS". As soon as an improvement is brought about on day one stop and see them two days later. As a matter of fact we now teach **"the rule of three".** On day one when treating a patient with marked pain and thus distress we only use our pain free techniques three times as a precaution. This way you cannot exacerbate a patient's condition. Too much enthusiasm can leave them sore the next day. We are all aware of the latent effects that any manual therapy may have. On subsequent visits you may choose to "SNAG" 10 times.

If no change is elicited then "SNAGS" are inappropriate. You expect an immediate improvement. Remember that other physiotherapy should also be given and as I stated in the introduction to Part One you should use the McKenzie approach when a patient has a Lumbar 4/5 lesion with a lateral shift.

In treating the cervical and upper thoracic spines with "SNAGS" the patient is seated on a chair. For the lumbar, middle and lower thoracic spines we require a plinth and a belt that can be adjusted in length. The belt needs to be 2.6 metres (8 feet) in length and made from car seatbelt material with a suitable easy to release clasp. As will become apparent it makes the patient stable while mobilisations with movement are carried out. The techniques will now be described as they would be applied for movements in the lumbar spine that are painful and/or restricted. When assessing your patients' active movements for restrictions and/or pain, you should do this in both sitting and standing. If their movement problems are only present when standing then "SNAGS" are only done in standing. If they have movement problems when sitting as well then your initial therapy would be in sitting and would progress to standing. They can also be applied with certain exercises. (See later) As with the cervical spine many patients, when taught, can apply "SELF SNAGS" and this will be covered at the end of this section.

Descriptions

(1). To increase flexion and/or decrease the pain associated with this movement.

a. In sitting

The patient sits on a plinth with his legs over the side. You stand behind and place a belt around him and yourself as shown in Figure 18a. In placing the belt around the patient's lower abdomen keep it below the anterior superior iliac spines for comfort. The belt should be below your hip joints. (Depends on your stature). The ulnar border of your right hand is now placed under the spinous process of the vertebra above at the suspected spinal segment. Your other hand should be placed on the bed to the left of the patient. The patient flexes forward until the pain is felt. He now backs off a little from this position. You now apply a gliding force with your right hand up along the

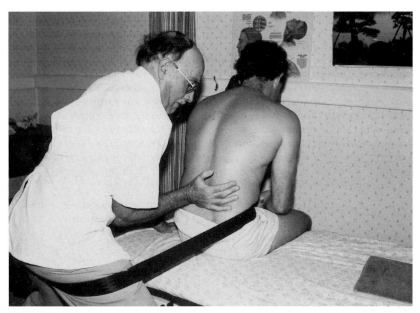

Figure 18a
"SNAGS" for lumbar flexion in sitting.

Figure 18b
"SNAGS" for lumbar flexion using thumbs over left lumbar 5 facet.

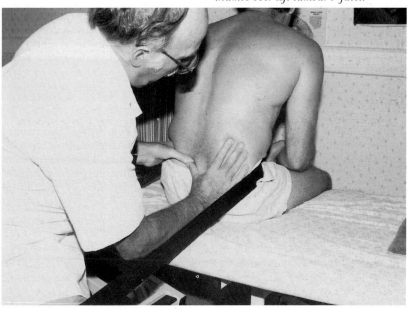

treatment plane as he again flexes. If the treatment is indicated, you are on the right segment and the direction of force is correct, he will painlessly flex to almost full range. If there is pain try another level. Sustain this flexed position for a few seconds and maintain your facet glide until the patient is again erect. Failure to maintain the glide could lead to a sharp and unnecessary pain. When there is no pain, repeat just three times and that would be all that you would do on the patient's first visit. If this central "SNAG" is not helpful a unilateral glide should be tried. Let us assume your patient has a Lumbar 4/5 segmental lesion. To do this place the ulnar border of your right hand (just distal to the pisaform) under the transverse process of Lumbar 4 on the right. As the patient flexes push up along the facet plane. If unsuccessful try a unilateral "SNAG" on the opposite side. With the passage of time I tend to use the unilateral "SNAG" rather than the central.

Instead of the ulnar border of the hand, the thumbs are used when dealing with the lumbosacral level unilaterally. As with the cervical spine one thumb reinforces the other which is placed over the superior facet.(See figure 18b). They glide the superior Lumbar 5 facet up on the sacral facet as flexion takes place. N.B. It is impossible to use your thumbs above the lumbo/sacral segment as the inferior facet projects posteriorly further than its partner making correct thumb contact impossible.

Important

When treating a patient who presents with an acute lumbar lesion and responds immediately to flexion "SNAGS" , stop after three repetitions and tape the spine in hyperextension to prevent further aggravation. Two strips of 2.5 centimetre adhesive tape used diagonally across the lumbar spine are extremely effective. We would of course encourage extensions as they would be taught by physiotherapists using R A McKenzie's protocols. At this juncture I would add one proviso and that is we would avoid extension if it was painful.

b. In standing

With the patient standing, place the now familiar belt around the patient and yourself as it was when the patient was seated. (See figure 18c). "SNAGS" are now undertaken in the same way as they were in sitting. However have the patient slightly flex his knees as this will remove hamstring and neural tension facilitating a better response. Remember as with all "SNAGS" techniques maintain your pressure until the patient is erect again. It may be necessary to "SNAG" unilaterally as suggested when the patient is sitting and this is done in exactly the same way. The patients' response is often improved if they are close to a table or bed on which they can place a hand for stability.

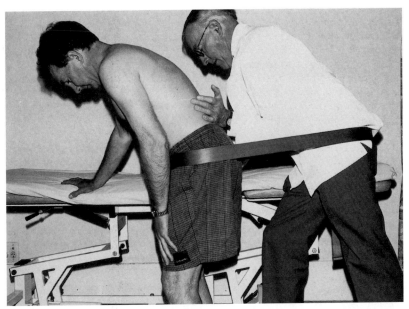

Figure 18c
"SNAGS" for lumbar flexion in standing.

(2). To increase extension and/or decrease the pain associated with this movement.

If extension is painful and limited in sitting then you would start with the patient sitting on the plinth with his legs over the side. You stand behind the patient with the belt around you both. I find it easier to have it lower on me as you will see in Figure 19a. The ulnar border of your right (or left) hand is placed under the superior spinous process of the vertebral segment involved. Providing he feels no pain the patient extends his lumbar spine while you push up along the treatment plane. If you study the photograph of this technique you will note that I am standing to the side of the patient to ensure I am not in way as he extends. His co-operation is essential. If painful he must stop and you would try another level. If still painful try "SNAGGING" over the transverse process on the right or perhaps the left.

N.B. A problem encountered with some patients is that they lean back against your hand instead of extending their lumbar spines. This is terrible as you take all the upper body weight and feel that your wrist may break. See that they get it right!

We all see many patients with chronic low back pain who on examination have painful limited extension and apparent normal pain free flexion. What is often necessary with these sufferers if "SNAGS" for extension is unsuccess-

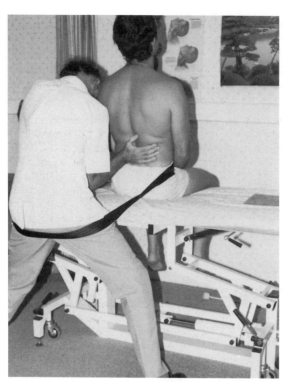

Figure 19a

"SNAGS" for lumbar extension in sitting.

Figure 19b

"SNAGS" for lumbar extension in standing

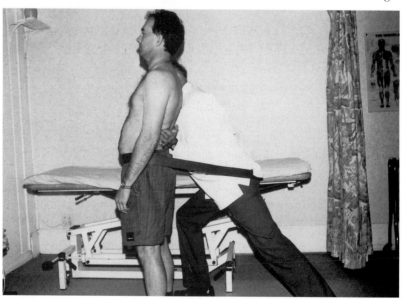

Manual Therapy

ful, is to "SNAG" them in flexion first. This would appear to release the facet(s) at the offending level and make a spectacular difference when "SNAGS" are again repeated for extension.

As with the "SNAGS" technique for flexion you would progress to the standing position. Standing would of course be the starting position if extension in sitting was symptomless in the first place. (See figure 19b)

When "SNAGS" for extension are indicated repeat the mobilisation with movement only three times on day one. The patient should now be able to extend unassisted and without pain. More "SNAGS" may be required but do not over treat on day one . Some patients feel discomfort the next day but if the rules with regard to pain are followed no problems will be encountered. If the articular pillar on one side is being chosen for extension, select the side of pain first. This technique can be a strain on the therapist. To minimise this, tuck the elbow of the mobilising arm into your waist and keep the leg on this side well behind you for stability.

QUESTION?

When teaching "SNAGS" for extension, physiotherapists often ask for an explanation as to why I glide the superior facet up for extension when it biomechanically is supposed to slide down. One theory I hesitantly offer is that the superior facet is 'jammed' down on its partner and extension 'jams' it further. Pushing it up before extension takes place re- positions it to enable it to now behave biomechanically as it was designed to. I guess the point is they work when indicated and that is all that matters.

(3). To increase rotation and/or decrease the pain associated with this movement

The patient sits astride one end of the plinth facing the other end. This stabilises the pelvis which is important. He places his hands behind his neck. Let us assume the patient has a painful loss of right rotation resulting from a lesion at the Lumbar 2/3 level. You stand at his right side and wrap your right arm around him clasping the side just above the suspected level of the lesion. (See figure 20). The ulnar border of your left hand is placed under the spinous process of Lumbar 2. The patient now rotates to the right as your left hand "SNAGS" the segment. There must be no pain. Your right hand around the waist encourages the movement and will apply overpressure at end range. To this end your hand around the waist must be above the level of the segment being treated or it will be unable to apply overpressure. If this procedure is ineffective you can next try "SNAGS" over the transverse process on the right or left. To do this use the ulnar border of the hand just distal to the pisaform to effect the glide. If the elbow of the mobilising arm rests in the ventral fold of your hip joint then an upward glide of your pelvis will assist with the facet glide. It should produce no pain.

D. THE SACRO ILIAC (S/I) JOINTS

Is there something enigmatic about these joints? I ask this because they are completely ignored by some authorities on back pain and dealt with in unbelievable detail by others. The omission by the former is bewildering as can be the details of the latter.

My approach is simplistic, effective when indicated, and when it has no place then a greater depth of knowledge is required. I do know that often the patient has a leg length discrepancy and I would supply them with a heel raise, cut from carpet, to address this and see if this is advantageous. I do know that weightbearing can be a problem. Walking can exacerbate their symptoms whereas patients with a lumbar lesion are usually more comfortable on their feet. They often have leg pain mimicking a 'disc' but their SLR is normal.

Actually, I do not wish to go through all the signs and symptoms attributed to S/I problems. However I would suggest that as a readable good source of information read what J.E.Bourdillon says about these joints in his book "Spinal Manipulation". He describes two 'positional faults' encountered in the S/I joints that can cause pain. One is called the 'posterior innonimate' where the ilium is slightly backwards on its sacral facet and the other is the opposite called the 'anterior innonimate' positioning and yes, there is a rotation component. These terms are osteopathic in origin. He claims that one is more likely to encounter the 'posterior innonimate' fault and I would agree.

The joint is so often troublesome during pregnancy because of the ligamentous laxity of the pelvic structures. A firm S/I support can be very useful to these patients and of course to others when instability is a factor.

When examining patients with back and/or leg pain I always do a spring test on the lumbar segments and on the posterior border of the ilium to see if it produces pain. When a sacro-iliac joint is involved you will usually find that it is only pressure on the ilium that is painful.

Description

The posterior innonimate

If you suspect that the patient has a right posterior innonimate problem and they have pain with back extension in standing and/or lying, as well as with the spring test try this "Mobilisation with Movement".

The patient is lying prone. Stand to the left side of him and place the thenar eminence of your right hand on the slightly protruding posterior border of the right ilium and push it away from you (laterally). This should produce no pain. Now have the patient do a passive extension in lying, 'a la McKenzie', (half press-up) provided there is no pain. (See figure 23a) Repeat 10 times and if the procedure is indicated they should now extend with much less pain. Up

ful, is to "SNAG" them in flexion first. This would appear to release the facet(s) at the offending level and make a spectacular difference when "SNAGS" are again repeated for extension.

As with the "SNAGS" technique for flexion you would progress to the standing position. Standing would of course be the starting position if extension in sitting was symptomless in the first place. (See figure 19b)

When "SNAGS" for extension are indicated repeat the mobilisation with movement only three times on day one. The patient should now be able to extend unassisted and without pain. More "SNAGS" may be required but do not over treat on day one . Some patients feel discomfort the next day but if the rules with regard to pain are followed no problems will be encountered. If the articular pillar on one side is being chosen for extension, select the side of pain first. This technique can be a strain on the therapist. To minimise this, tuck the elbow of the mobilising arm into your waist and keep the leg on this side well behind you for stability.

QUESTION?

When teaching "SNAGS" for extension, physiotherapists often ask for an explanation as to why I glide the superior facet up for extension when it biomechanically is supposed to slide down. One theory I hesitantly offer is that the superior facet is 'jammed' down on its partner and extension 'jams' it further. Pushing it up before extension takes place re- positions it to enable it to now behave biomechanically as it was designed to. I guess the point is they work when indicated and that is all that matters.

(3). To increase rotation and/or decrease the pain associated with this movement

The patient sits astride one end of the plinth facing the other end. This stabilises the pelvis which is important. He places his hands behind his neck. Let us assume the patient has a painful loss of right rotation resulting from a lesion at the Lumbar 2/3 level. You stand at his right side and wrap your right arm around him clasping the side just above the suspected level of the lesion. (See figure 20). The ulnar border of your left hand is placed under the spinous process of Lumbar 2. The patient now rotates to the right as your left hand "SNAGS" the segment. There must be no pain. Your right hand around the waist encourages the movement and will apply overpressure at end range. To this end your hand around the waist must be above the level of the segment being treated or it will be unable to apply overpressure. If this procedure is ineffective you can next try "SNAGS" over the transverse process on the right or left. To do this use the ulnar border of the hand just distal to the pisiform to effect the glide. If the elbow of the mobilising arm rests in the ventral fold of your hip joint then an upward glide of your pelvis will assist with the facet glide. It should produce no pain.

(4). To increase side flexion and/or decrease the pain associated with this movement.

"SNAGS" are really useful for a side flexion loss. Even if you have a patient with a lateral shift that is proving recalcitrant try restoring side flexion in the manner to be described. The patient sits on the side of the bed with his back to you. A belt is around you both as demonstrated in Figure 20. For a loss of right side flexion, place the ulnar border of your right hand over the appropriate spinous process as has now been described many times. You would stand to the left of the patient. The belt would then serve to stabilise the patient as he side flexes while you are gliding the superior facet up. Active pain free movement can be expected if the technique is correct and you have chosen the correct level. You could repeat this mobilisation with movement three times and that would be sufficient on the first visit.

This technique can be applied in standing if thought necessary though it is more difficult on the operator.

As with all the previous treatments that have been covered you may have to "SNAG" over a transverse process. The transverse process on the painful side would be my first choice.

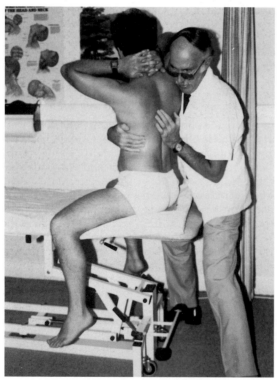

Figure 20

"SNAGS" for lumbar or thoracic rotation in sitting

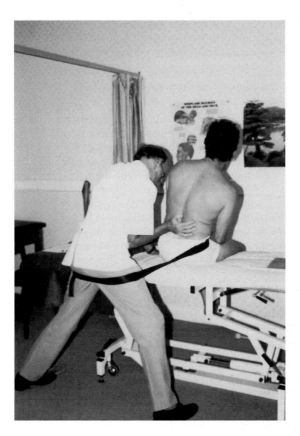

Figure 21
"SNAGS" for lumbar
side flexion in sitting.

2. "SELF SNAGS"

Explanation and Description

As with the cervical spine it is possible for many patients to "SELF SNAG" their lumbar spines particularly for flexion and extension and sometimes for side flexion. They can be great. I would like here to refer to the repeated extensions in standing recommended by McKenzie. These are encouraged for instance if they centralise a pain that is experienced in the posterior thigh. When a belt is used successfully by the patient to "SELF SNAG" they can do repeated extensions in standing painlessly and after several repetitions actively extend without the belt painlessly. The purpose of "SNAGS" is to bring about an immediate improvement in the patient's movement after they have been completed. To successfully "SNAG" a joint several times and find that there is no change following their application would suggest that the treatment is inappropriate.

The patient requires a belt, (ideally of car seat belt material or soft leather), that is long enough to pass around his back and still be held at short arm's length away from his body on each side. (See figure 22a). My wife can "SELF SNAG" using the selvage of a bath towel.

If the segmental lesion is at Lumbar 3/4 then the belt is hooked under the spinous process of Lumbar 3.

Extension is the most commonly used "SELF SNAG". The patient pulls up on the belt in the direction of his chin and moves into spinal extension if no pain is experienced. This is repeated say ten times and then two hourly or as you think necessary. Another method is to have the patient clench a fist and place the shaft of the first phalanx of his index finger under the spinous process. With the assistance of his other hand he pushes up along the treatment plane as he extends. For unilateral "SELF SNAGS" again a fist is used. This time the flexed metacarpo-phalangeal joint of the index finger is placed over the transverse process on one side. (See figure 22b). As said before an articulated spine is a wonderful asset to use when trying to explain to a patient where to push and of course to explain what the technique is all about.

It helps if the patient is intelligent and has reasonably strong arms.

"SELF SNAGS" for flexion are accomplished in the same way as for extension. However as with "SNAGS" have the patient slightly flex his knees to ease the tension on the hamstrings and neural tissue.

Warning. If flexion is limited and the patient is in a great deal of pain, "SELF SNAGS" for flexion would be inadvisable until with your management they feel more comfortable.

N.B. Sometimes when an extension "SELF SNAG" appears to be ineffective try a flexion "SELF SNAG" first and then extend. This can be very spectacular with really painful backs and when gross restrictions are present. I presume that the offending facets are too 'jammed' to be influenced when an extension "SELF SNAG" is applied and that by flexing first it frees the facet so that painless extension can now occur. Therapists on my courses have witnessed this ever so often. In their presence we would get the patient to do repeated flexion/extension "SELF SNAGS" and each attempt would see a progressive improvement.

The common fault, that we encounter with "SELF SNAGS", is when the patient fails to maintain the pull up along the treatment plane as the movement takes place. He starts off correctly but forgets to keep pulling up towards his chin as he goes back. Another problem is that he releases the pull up before he returns to the upright position. "SELF SNAGS" with a belt for the lumbo-sacral joint will not work if the patient's posterior iliac borders protrude further posteriorly than Lumbar 5's spinous process. The edge of the belt cannot physically make contact with it.

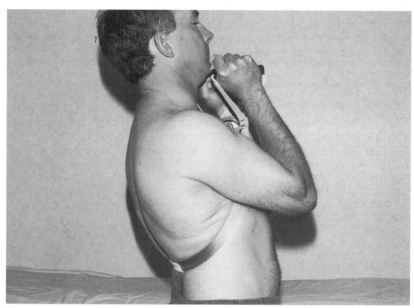

Figure 22a
"SELF SNAGS" for lumbar extension using a belt.

Figure 22b
"SELF SNAGS" for lumbar extension using hands.

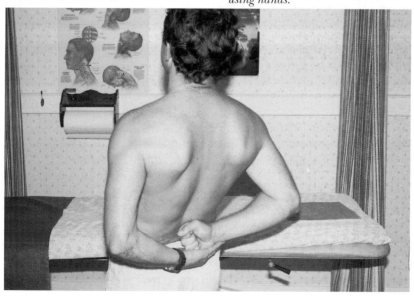

D. THE SACRO ILIAC (S/I) JOINTS

Is there something enigmatic about these joints? I ask this because they are completely ignored by some authorities on back pain and dealt with in unbelievable detail by others. The omission by the former is bewildering as can be the details of the latter.

My approach is simplistic, effective when indicated, and when it has no place then a greater depth of knowledge is required. I do know that often the patient has a leg length discrepancy and I would supply them with a heel raise, cut from carpet, to address this and see if this is advantageous. I do know that weightbearing can be a problem. Walking can exacerbate their symptoms whereas patients with a lumbar lesion are usually more comfortable on their feet. They often have leg pain mimicking a 'disc' but their SLR is normal.

Actually, I do not wish to go through all the signs and symptoms attributed to S/I problems. However I would suggest that as a readable good source of information read what J.E.Bourdillon says about these joints in his book "Spinal Manipulation". He describes two 'positional faults' encountered in the S/I joints that can cause pain. One is called the 'posterior innominate' where the ilium is slightly backwards on its sacral facet and the other is the opposite called the 'anterior innominate' positioning and yes, there is a rotation component. These terms are osteopathic in origin. He claims that one is more likely to encounter the 'posterior innominate' fault and I would agree.

The joint is so often troublesome during pregnancy because of the ligamentous laxity of the pelvic structures. A firm S/I support can be very useful to these patients and of course to others when instability is a factor.

When examining patients with back and/or leg pain I always do a spring test on the lumbar segments and on the posterior border of the ilium to see if it produces pain. When a sacro-iliac joint is involved you will usually find that it is only pressure on the ilium that is painful.

Description

The posterior innominate

If you suspect that the patient has a right posterior innominate problem and they have pain with back extension in standing and/or lying, as well as with the spring test try this "Mobilisation with Movement".

The patient is lying prone. Stand to the left side of him and place the thenar eminence of your right hand on the slightly protruding posterior border of the right ilium and push it away from you (laterally). This should produce no pain. Now have the patient do a passive extension in lying, 'a la McKenzie',(half press-up) provided there is no pain. (See figure 23a) Repeat 10 times and if the procedure is indicated they should now extend with much less pain. Up

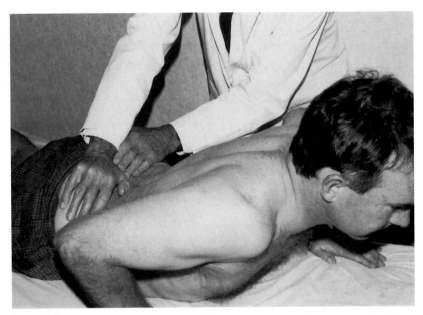

Figure 23a

"MWM" Sacro-iliac joint; posterior innonimate.

to three sets of 10 can given bearing in mind the effort required. Some subtle variations in your thenar placement and in the lateral direction should be tried if there is discomfort. Subtle handling and directional changes are true of all MWM techniques.

Many patients with back pain have a positive 'spring test' sign but can extend without pain. Still use this technique as you will often find after three sets of 10 this positive sign has gone. In many instances I have brought in the partners of patients and shown them where to push so that the patient can have further MWMS at home between visits. I will often suggest that the partner 'treats' her/his mate two or three times a day to speed up the recovery.

The anterior innonimate

About four years ago two of my accredited teachers, Peter van Dalen and Rene Claassen, said they had had success with some sacroiliac problems by having the patient extend his spine standing, while they fixated the sacrum with one hand and pulled back on the ilium on the offending side with other. How logical. This is really the opposite of what I have described above and would be used for the anterior innonimate fault. However I will start by describing how you would treat the patient in lying.

The patient lies prone and you stand at his side, opposite to the lesion. Fixate the sacrum with the border of one hand and place the fingers of your other hand under the right anterior superior iliac spine if the right S/I is involved. Pull up the ilium on the sacrum and hold this position while the patient does 10 half press-ups, provided these are pain free. Two further sets of 10 may now be done. (See figure 23b)

As mentioned these could be done in standing, as suggested by my colleagues, if in standing extension was painful. If pelvic tilting was painful in standing have the patient do this while you hold the ilium and sacrum in the same way.

Often patients have S/I pain walking. If you suspect an anterior innonimate, stand behind them and use the hand placement for prone lying. Now with the ilium held back have them walk. When indicated they will walk with no pain. I have, when teaching on my courses, had patients stroll up and down a ballroom with me holding on in the above manner. I am sure I look quite ridiculous to the onlooker as I follow behind. It makes me puff a little but I come to no harm. When this is successful you can tape the patient. Begin with the 5cm wide tape in front of the anterior superior iliac spine and wrap it around obliquely to terminate over the lumbar spine.

As a manipulative therapist I have the option to manipulate this joint but this can sometimes be difficult to do with some patients for a variety of reasons, so it is nice to have the above MWMS .

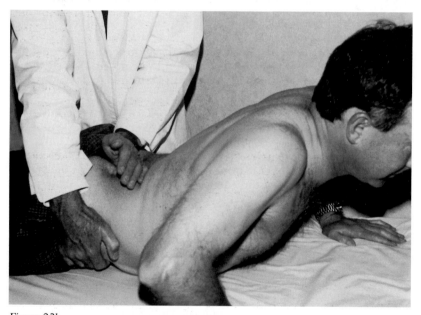

Figure 23b

"MWM" Sacro-iliac joint; anteror innonimate.

E. THE THORACIC SPINE

"SNAGS"

Explanation and Descriptions

As the reader would expect the techniques for the thoracic spine are really the same as those for the lumbar spine. In practice the most useful "SNAG" is the one for rotation as this is the movement most commonly requiring attention in patients with thoracic lesions.

(1). To restore rotation and/or decrease the pain associated with this movement

The patient positioning and technique is the same as that for lumbar rotation. If you refer back to figure 20 you will note that the patient's hands are behind the neck. This is done to move the scapulae away from the vertebrae to make the latter more accessible. It is difficult with large patients particularly women. The problem, if you have short arms, comes when you try to wrap your arm around the patient to clasp the side just above the suspected level.

Experience will show you that unilateral positioning is required more frequently than central positioning over the spinous process. Do not over "SNAG". As soon as a marked improvement is obtained, stop. Quite often with thoracic lesions you need to deal with both right and left rotation and you would do this on day one if both were involved. After restoring pain free rotation I always then support the thoracic spine for 48 hours with two short pieces of 5 centimetre wide zinc oxide tape, placed diagonally across the site of the lesion.

Sometimes following a successful "SNAG" minor movement discomfort may be encountered at another level. It is easily dealt with. Treat this as above. I tell my patients their spines just require some fine tuning.

(2). To restore flexion and/or decrease the pain associated with this movement

The patient sits astride the plinth as for rotation. If you are standing behind and to his right, place your right arm around his trunk at the level of the lesion. This is used as a fulcrum for bending. Your left hand's ulnar border is placed over the selected spinous process or the transverse process and supplies the gliding force along the facet plane as the patient flexes. (See Figure 24)

(3). To restore extension and/or decrease the pain associated with it

In the lower thoracic spine the "SNAGS" procedure is the same as that used for the lumbar spine. (i.e. belt)

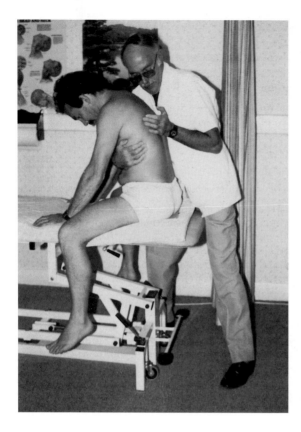

Figure 24

"SNAGS" to restore flexion in thoracic spine.

For the mid thoracic spine the patient sits astride the plinth with you at his side. As you will see from Figure 25 one hand is applying the "SNAGS" while the free arm is wrapped around the patient guiding the movement. Some strength is required to support the patient during extension as well as providing the facet glide. It is easier to have the flexed elbow of the arm responsible for the "SNAGS" tucked into your side. This would be the most physically demanding of all the "SNAGS" techniques. Thank goodness that this technique is rarely required. As already stated rotation techniques are generally used in the thoracic spine.

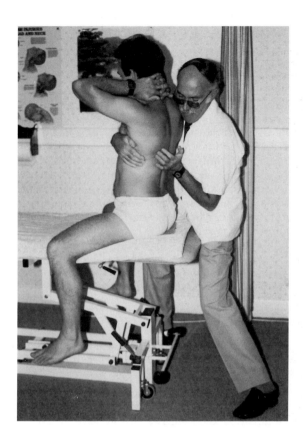

Figure 25
"SNAGS" to restore ex-
tension in thoracic
spine.

F. THE RIB CAGE

As ' Mobilisations with Movement' had proved successful in the spine (SNAGS) and most certainly in the extremity joints I guess it was inevitable that I would try them on the rib cage. Yes the MWM procedures can be very successful and I would invite you to add them to your therapies for chest wall pain with movement. I mean skeletal pain that does not appear to be of spinal origin and certainly not from heart, lung or other pathologies. The pain producing movements may be rotation, side flexion, flexion, extension or combinations of these or perhaps deep breathing. All of these can come directly from a spinal lesion but you must not discount rib cage dysfunction as a possible source of the above symptoms. Like all other MWM techniques it can quickly be ascertained if a rib MWM is a value. When applying Thoracic SNAGS unilaterally over a transverse process, it is impossible to exclude the costo-vertebral joints because of your hand positioning. This might, in no small measure, explain why the SNAGS can be so successful when other manual therapy procedures such as mobilisation and manipulation have failed. This led me to experiment on patients with anterior, lateral, antero or postero-lateral chest pain by SNAGGING the rib cage.

Examples

A patient experiences right anterior chest pain with right rotation that has not responded to spinal techniques.

The patient sits astride at one end of your plinth, facing the other end. To move the scapulae away from the thoracic spinous processes have his hands clasped behind his neck. Stand at the right side of him and place the medial border of your right hand (sloping) along the inferior border of the chosen rib, to lift it and separate it from its neighbour. (Remember that the ribs lie like bucket handles thus lying slightly obliquely in front and behind and more or less horizontally laterally. The chondral components of the ribs coming laterally from the sternum are virtually horizontal.) Your other hand is placed on the posterior chest wall (sloping) positioned as in front. Lift the rib up with both hands and have the patient carry out the offending rotation. If pain free, use your hands so positioned to apply some overpressure. (see figure 26a) I sometimes get a colleague to apply rotation overpressure.

When indicated and pain free rotation occurs, the patient should feel much better after 6-10 repetitions.

How do you know which rib to be on? If anteriorly the space between the 6th and 7th ribs is painful then lift the 6th. Sometimes trial and error is needed. Always ask the patient to move cautiously and stop if there is any discomfort. Following the rules for MWMS is foolproof. The technique is contra indicated if it cannot be undertaken without symptoms.

The same positioning could be used for rib cage pain with flexion or extension.

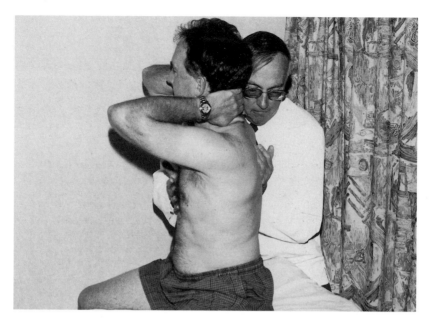

Figure 26a

"SNAGS" to the rib cage with rotation.

Very common indeed is sterno-costal pain following strenuous exercise. The patient usually complains of localised pain with thoracic extension or horizontal extension of the arm on the affected side. With hand placement as above have the patient extend . If pain free you will notice an immediate improvement in function after perhaps just one or two MWMS.

With female patients who have anterior rib pain beneath a breast, careful hand placement is required to make painless contact with a rib and with too much breast tissue the technique may not be possible. (See figure 26b) I used this technique successfully on a therapist last year who was unable to rotate her trunk to the right for three years because of pain under her right breast. It was really spectacular and the result was witnessed by a large class.

Lateral chest pain of rib origin is dealt with by standing behind the patient seated as above and placing one hand along and under the chosen rib to lift it as the patient side flexes. The other hand would be on the chest wall laterally on the opposite side.

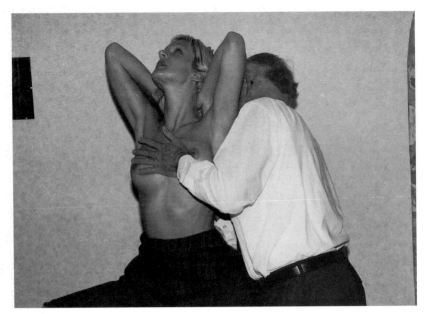

Figure 26b
"SNAGS" for anterior chest pain with extension.

The 1st and 2nd ribs

When these are involved, patients often experience pain along the trapezius muscle between the neck and shoulder when side flexing away from the side of pain.

Stand behind the patient, fixate the first (or second) rib antero-laterally with one hand while you apply overpressure with your other hand to the head after the patient has side flexed away. when this is indicated there is no pain after repetitions, they should be pain free. I use the radial border of the mc/p joint of my index finger over the rib to fixate as shown in figure 26c.

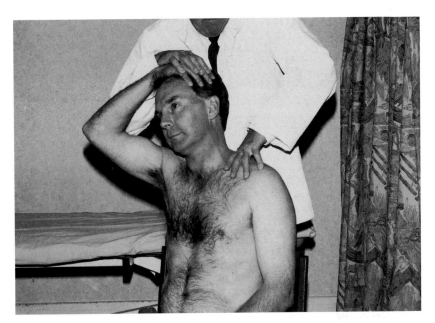

Figure 26c

"SNAGS" for 1st rib with side flexion.

G. CONCLUSION

All the "NAGS" and "SNAGS" techniques described in this section on the spine are basic ones. Once they are mastered therapists adapt them to their own requirements. This may be necessary because of different body types. I use many starting variations but the principles are not altered. Some patients present with more than one level of involvement and this requires some imagination to deal with. I have even combined them with a slump stretch and when next you get a patient with a limited straight leg raise, and apparent normal spinal movement, "SNAG" for flexion over Lumbar 5 or perhaps Lumbar 4 and see what happens when you retest. When next you have a patient with a persistent hamstring lesion try a lumbo-sacral "SNAGS" and see if this "fixes" the problem.

One difficulty encountered but easily solved is due to perspiration particularly in hot climates. If either the patient's or your skin is moist then slipping will occur particularly with "SNAGS". This can be overcome by the use of a paper tissue. (e.g. Kleenex or Snowtex)

If you abide by the rules no complications will arise and remember, do not do too much on the patient's first visit.

H. COURSE HANDOUTS

1.
CERVICAL SPINE : GUIDELINES AS TO WHICH TECHNIQUE TO USE

MOBILISATIONS ONLY

Firstly there are already indications as to when to use mobilisations from the teachings of manual therapists Maitland, Kaltenborn etc.

NAGS are used to restore movement and because of the no pain concept are particularly useful in

1. The elderly.
2. With the acute neck presenting with a gross loss of movement.
3. As a test for irritability. (if one is not able to NAG without pain then beware of all forms of manual therapy)

REVERSE NAGS bilaterally or unlaterally are super for..

1. Those patients with end range losses of neck movement.
2. For computer or desk related neck pain due to the poor forward projecting neck posture.
3. Degenerative lower cervical/upper thoracic spines etc.

FIST TRACTIONS

For a loss of lower Cervical flexion

MOBILISATIONS AND/OR MOBILISATIONS WITH MOVEMENT

TWO MAIN CATEGORIES.
1. Neck Pain And Stiffness With No Arm Involvement.
a. NAGS cervical spine
b. REVERSE NAGS upper thoracic and lower cervical spines
c. MWMs segmentally (i.e. Cx5/6) with active rotation, flexion, extension
d. SNAGS and SELF SNAGS with rotation, side flexion , extension
2. Neck Pain And Stiffness With Arm Involvement.
a. When arm movement causes neck pain only. MWM for non radicular pain from Cx 5/6 experienced with right shoulder abduction would be Cx 5 spinous process to left with right abduction.

b. When arm movement causes arm pain of cervical origin. MWM for pain referred to right thumb with right abduction would be Cx5 spinous process to left with right abduction.

c. With both examples given above you may ask the patient to move concurrently the head to the right, (with overpressure), with the arm when using this MWM.

PS REMEMBER WITH ALL THE ABOVE TECHNIQUES THERE WOULD BE NO PAIN . NO PAIN IS THE PRIME INDICATION FOR THEIR USE.

2.

LUMBAR EXERCISES

1. Passive Back extensions:

Lie on your front with hands placed next to your chest. Keeping your hips in contact with the ground, push your chest off the ground as far as possible (with no pain), then return to starting position.

If pain is experienced, place hands closer to waist level and repeat.

For one sided pain with this exercise place a pillow under your hip on that side

Stop if pain persists.

REPEAT 10X

2. Lion exercises:

On all fours kneeling, place knees wider apart than shoulders, keeping arms straight and hands stationary, move your buttocks back towards feet. Return to starting position.

REPEAT 10X

Alternatives:

a. If painful, either hollow your lower back and repeat above, or hump lower back and repeat.

b. If pain is more one sided , place knee on that side slightly closer to hands than the other. When moving backwards ensure you go straight back and not veer to the side.

c. For one sided pain with this exercise place pad under knee on side of pain and then move your buttocks towards your feet

2. OTHER SPINAL THERAPIES

A. Manipulation

I would support those who claim that manipulations are much more useful in the treatment programs for the cervical and upper thoracic spines than in the management of lumbar and lower thoracic lesions. This is because the facet joints are probably more directly responsible for pain emanating from the cervical spine. Physiotherapists should read "Where Is The Pain Coming From" by V. Mooney published in "Spine" in 1987.

In my preamble on "SNAGS' at the beginning of the section on the lumbar spine I wrote of the need to have mobile facets for normal discal distortions to take place with spinal movement. What happens when we manipulate a lumbar spinal joint? We hear and feel a click. Most practitioners agree that this is usually a facet sound. Some patients feel instantly better but others say it has made no difference even though you are sure the correct segment has been dealt with. I would say with the former the manipulation has enabled the facet joints to glide normally removing the abnormal strain on the disc. With the latter the joints, though manipulatively gapped, are still unable to perform normally. To use "SNAGS" makes sense but there are patients who fail to respond to these but will do so after a preceding manipulation. The danger from manipulation as I see it is from manipulating with the "wrong side up". Strict guidelines cannot be given. If the incorrect side is chosen too much unnatural torsion strain can be placed on a weakened disc. It is not until after your manipulation that you find you have worsened the disc pathology. Dangers are minimised by skilled manipulators who, because of their technical ability, use minimal force when thrusting. However "SNAGS" are much safer.

B. Belt traction techniques

The belt I use for "SNAGS" to the lumbar spine and adequately described in earlier text can be used to apply traction to many segments of the spine. I had an article published on this subject in Gregory Grieve's magnificent tome "Modern Manual Therapy of the Vertebral column".

In the preface I mentioned how techniques change for the better as time passes. This is certainly true of a technique described in my paper in Greg Grieve's book. It relates to the application of traction to the middle and lower thoracic and lumbar spines. Although, as explained, it achieves a successful distraction the strain on the therapist is considerable. I have thus modified the procedure to avoid this and enable those of smaller stature to cope. The belt tractions for the cervical spine I have not had to alter.

For the mid-thoracic to the low lumbar spine have the patient lying supine on a plinth covered with non slip material. The plinth should be on carpeted floor to prevent it from moving when the patient is tractioned and be adjustable in height for convenience.

The belt is positioned under the spinous process of the vertebra above the offending segment and its loop encircles your shoulders. (See figure 27a). The patient needs to place his hands around your waist when dealing with the mid thoracic spine to move the scapulae laterally on the chest wall. A pillow may be placed under the head. The reader will see from Figure 27a that the therapist's hips are slightly flexed so that his trunk hovers over the patient's body. You place your hands on the plinth with bent arms. The hands will become a fulcrum for a movement about to take place. You now extend your arms to secure the belt at the chosen level and by leaning backwards and pivoting on the fully extended arms you will traction the spine distal to the belt. Making use of the arms in this way ensures that no stress is placed on your spine and this is important.

When traction like this is applied, stop when the patient starts to slide up the bed. Nothing further is achieved when this happens. A slightly stronger traction force can be applied if the patient parts his legs and drops his lower legs over the side. If he tries to cling to the sides of the bed with his legs positioned in this way it will achieve nothing as he must be relaxed for maximum benefit.

I have seen small therapists apply extremely effective traction on large patients without effort in this way.

The use of belts to apply traction to the vertebral column has introduced a hitherto unobtainable degree of specificity and make manual traction so easy.

Traction applied in this manner would be sustained for more than ten seconds and can be repeated and repeated over many minutes. If it produced

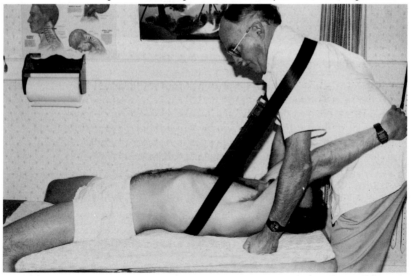

Figure 27a

Belt traction for thoracic or lumbar spine.

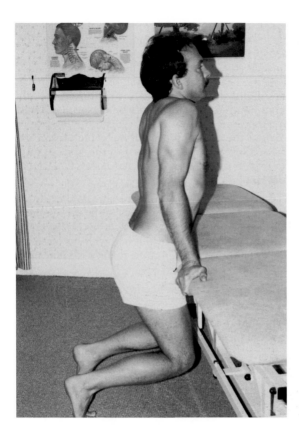

Figure 27b

*Self traction for the tho-
racic and lumbar
spines.*

any pain you would not use it. If a patient was experiencing thoracic pain with breathing it should not be present when the distraction is taking place and after several repetitions should have disappeared altogether. Patients with anterior thigh pain radiating from lumbar 2/3 should experience relief when traction is applied with the belt hooked on lumbar 2 (sometimes lumbar 1). Thoracic manipulations are much easier to do after traction has been locally applied. A good follow up home traction will be described next.

C. Self tractions for the mid and lower thoracic and lumbar spines

This technique can be invaluable for acute thoracic pain of spinal origin. With those patients who experience chest pain with breathing, relief is nearly always obtained. The procedure is simple and it is the time factor that makes it work.

The patient stands beside a table of suitable height. He places his hands on the table so that the distance between them is greater than the width of the hips. Keeping his elbows locked in extension he bends his knees and allows

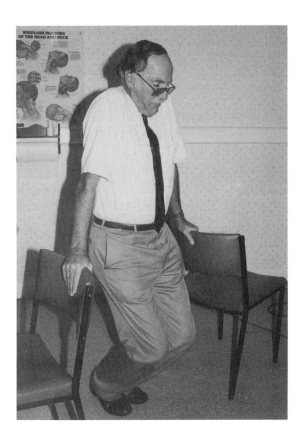

Figure 27c

Self traction for the thoracic spine between two chairs.

the body to sink. In this position the shoulders would be elevated, the flexed toes only would be on the floor and the front of the body would be against the table. Seen from the side, the head, shoulders and hips would be in a vertical line with the knees slightly forward of this. (See figure 27b). If the knees are placed behind the trunk, traction would not take place. Instead a form of extension would result and this would be useless.

Patients must maintain this position for at least 20 seconds. By this time any thoracic pain being experienced would have eased. If not, check the position to ensure it is correct. With the patients I spoke of with pain on inspiration, you should find that it has almost disappeared by the 20 seconds. If the correct technique does not relieve the pain then forget it. Try something else. In my practice I tell young patients that they are expected to self traction for 30 seconds three times and repeat this routine every two hours. Older patients are asked to self traction for 20 seconds three times and repeat this routine every two hours if they can manage it.

This form of self traction is a useful 'first aid' measure for patients smitten with sudden back pain.

Note! When standing up after self traction patients must take care not to flex the spine as this could spoil the therapy. To avoid this after the sustained traction they bring one foot forward so that it lies beneath them. They use this leg to stand straight up.

Another very good way of doing this is between the backs of two chairs. (See figure 27c) The hands clasp the adjacent chair backs and with the elbows straight bend you knees as above. It is hard on the palms of some patients and to get chair backs of suitable height is the other problem.

IMPORTANT!

The next four techniques to be described (D,E,F&G) are extremely important and are used daily in my practice, when Straight Leg Raising is involved, to see if one of them has a role to play as a treatment. In fact at least one of them is usually proved effective. The first three are used when the patient with limited SLR does not have any pain or signs below the knee. The fourth is used when the patient has pain and/or other signs radiating below the knee or a **positive femoral nerve** sign. The first two have the added advantage of being useful as a home treatment by the patient. I will discuss sitting later and a simple new chair design which modesty prevents me from saying is very very good.

D. The bent leg raise technique. (BLR)

This is a painless technique, when indicated, and can be tried on any patient with low back pain who has limited and/or painful straight leg raising (SLR). It can be tried even if they have leg pain above the knee and can be extremely useful when you are confronted with one of those patients who has a gross bilateral limitation of straight leg raising. You will never make them worse, if the absence of pain when applying your technique is your guide. If the bent leg raise (BLR) cannot be executed without pain then it is not to be used. The same rule as for "SNAGS". As with the techniques already covered in this book you do not over treat on the patient's first visit and we now teach the **'rule of three'** which means on day one the technique would only be used three times as a precaution against any latent exacerbation. We would try this technique on nearly every patient we see and it proves of great value with more than half of them. Remember it must not hurt.

You stand at the limited SLR side of the supine patient and if both sides are limited you stand at the side of greatest limitation.

We will firstly deal with the patient who has only a small loss or has a full but painful end range with SLR. You place his flexed knee over your shoulder as seen in Figure 28. You now ask him to push you away with his leg and then relax. At this point you push his bent knee up as far as you can in the direction of his shoulder on the same side provided there is no pain. If it is painful alter the direction by taking his leg more medially or laterally. Sustain this stretch for several seconds and then lower the leg to the bed. With the bent knee over your shoulder you include a traction component with this technique. When indicated the stretch does not hurt and after being repeated three times you expect a marked improvement when they again straight leg raise.

Let us now consider the patient with a gross loss of SLR but other neural signs. Maybe he can only SLR to 20 degrees. Place one hand under his knee and clasp under his heel with the other. You flex, and keep, his knee to 20 degrees and raise the heel just off the bed. The patient is now asked to push his leg down to the bed against your resistance and then relax. At this point you raise the leg gently as far as you can from the bed, maintaining or increasing the knee flexion and introducing some hip abduction at the same time. There must be no pain. If painful, alter the direction of the raise medially or laterally or even add some hip rotation. If still painful abandon the technique. As with the knee over your shoulder repeat three times and then reassess.

The patient can almost replicate the BLR technique, lying supine, by grasping his thigh posteriorly as close to the knee as possible and pulling up and out.

E. The two leg rotation technique, also known as the "gate" technique

This is another superb procedure for lumbar spine lesions that restrict straight leg raising. To me it is special because when useful it can be done successfully by the patient without assistance. For many years I would apply the technique but now I teach my patients to do it so that between visits they can carry on

Figure 28

The bent leg raise technique for the lumbar spine.

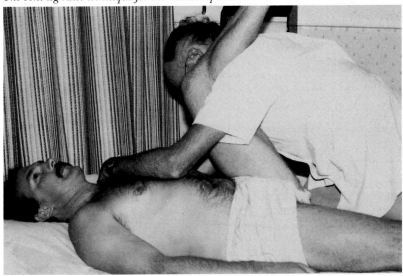

the therapy. It is always combined with other routines of course. It would never be done if it caused pain and initially, until it is established that it is going to be useful, it is done slowly and gently and the 'the rule of three' applies on the first visit.

Let us assume that our patient has limited straight leg raising on the right, and has no signs below the knee. He lies supine and grips the side of the plinth with his left hand. Both legs are now flexed so that the feet are off the plinth. Keeping his shoulders on the bed he takes his legs slowly to the side of the limited straight leg raise. (See figure 29a). He must feel no pain. If painful he alters the degree of flexion at the hips (more or less) to see if this enables further pelvic rotation. It usually will but he may again find further progress painful. If so, again alter the degree of flexion at the hips and see if further progress may be made with the rotation. When he reaches his limit the position is sustained for several seconds before returning to a crook lying position. He then places first one leg and then the other out straight on the bed. At this point SLR is measured. In nearly every case when the technique can be undertaken painlessly you will see an improvement. The whole process is repeated another two times when further progress will have been made.

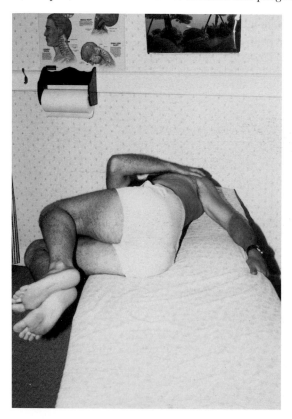

Figure 29a

The two leg rotation or "gate" technique.

The patient is then instructed to repeat the treatment at regular intervals as you think fit.

This technique can be called the "gate technique" for the following reason. When the patient attempts to take his knees to the side of the limited straight leg raise the movement may stop as if he has encountered a barrier like a fence. By increasing or decreasing his hip flexion, further movement takes place as if he has found a gate in the fence and gone through it. He again may encounter a further barrier (fence) and with altered hip flexion [finds the next 'gate' to go through and so on. If he cannot find a 'gate' then pain will warn you that the treatment is not appropriate.

Difficulties? There are two problems that you will encounter

The first is apprehension. Some patients with very sore backs are very apprehensive of this technique. Let them measure and note their straight leg raise limitation and then coax them to gently try the technique but do not go too far. Return them to the starting position and let them remeasure their SLR. If it has visibly improved their attitude to the next rotation will be free from any apprehension.

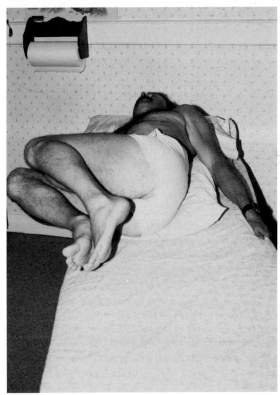

Figure 29b

The "gate" technique off two pillows.

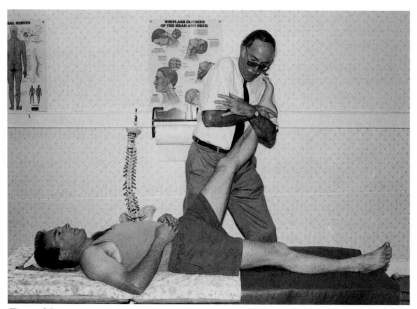

Figure 30

Straight leg raise with traction.

The second is the bed on which they try to do their own two leg rotations. When using the plinth in your clinic they are normally able to rotate to a position where their knees are over the side of the bed. At home they are restricted when a wide bed is used. We suggest that they place two pillows longways under the trunk to raise it higher than the mattress. Figure 29b

F. (i) Straight leg raise with traction

The reason given in many texts as to why there is pain (with or without limitation) on straight leg raising is because nerve tissue is being stretched over an obstruction. This could not be the case when SLR with traction proves successful. However I will let you, the reader, be the judge of this. For this technique to work it is necessary that the patient can SLR to at least 40 degrees and his symptoms are above the knee. We have been able, using this procedure, to improve the status of patients who have failed to respond to other therapies delivered by all sorts of manual therapy practitioners.

Let us assume we have a patient who has right SLR loss which ,at the end of his available range, produces a referred pain to his right posterior thigh. The patient is supine and you stand facing his right side. You get him to actively SLR without your assistance and you both note the range. You now grasp his lower leg proximal to the ankle joint and raise it off the bed to a position just short of the painful range. Flex your knees and hold the clasped leg to your chest. When you extend your knees this will effectively apply a longitudinal traction to the leg provided the bed is low enough and you are tall enough. (See figure 30) Sustain this traction and undertake a straight leg raise as far as it will go provided there is no pain. If there is pain you may find that it disappears if you slightly rotate, abduct or adduct the hip as you raise the leg. When pain free, SLR with traction three times and watch as the patient reassesses his SLR. There should be smiles all round.

When successful you may on subsequent visits do more than three repetitions and use over pressure provided there is no discomfort. To SLR with traction painlessly in this manner must surely defy the textbook rationale already mentioned.

Remember that the technique is only part of the therapy.

(ii) Straight leg raise with 'compression'.

This technique is the opposite to the above in that instead of distracting the leg while you straight leg raise, you do the opposite.

You stand to the side of the supine patient and grasp the patient's straight leg to you body just short of the painful range.(see figure 31) Now apply a force along the long axis of the leg and slowly try to SLR provided there is no pain. To do this, varying degrees of hip abduction should be added in an endeavour to find a pain free pathway. In applying your 'compression' component

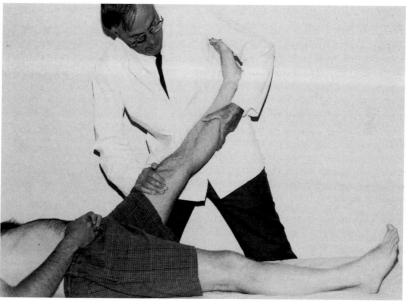

Figure 31
Straight leg raise with "compression"

ensure that your hand placement prevents the knee from flexing. When indicated, the end result is a marked improvement in the patient's active SLR. Remember three only repetitions on day one but on subsequent visits more can be given.

The success of such a procedure may be due to a lateral pressure being applied to a disc causing the 'bulge' to reduce and allow the leg movement to occur. Who knows?

Tight hamstrings?

Observers have noted that many patients with recurring low back pain appear to have tight hamstrings. Try straight leg raise with traction and you may be surprised at the rapid increase in the range of movement. You would never get the same result with a conventional hamstring stretch.

I often see patients who present with a chronic "hamstring strain" . The SLR is reduced and when you use the SLR with traction technique their problem is resolved in just a few treatments.

G. Spinal Mobilisations with Leg Movement. (SMWLM'S)

This technique would be my first choice when a patient presents with a lumbar lesion resulting in pain and other signs below the knee. I have already stated that the three previous techniques would be used when the signs and symptoms do not involve the lower leg. It would also be my choice with patients presenting with a **positive Femoral Nerve Sign.**

In part one of this book, sub-section 5., "Spinal Mobilisations with Arm Movement" were dealt with. Chronologically in my voyages of discovery in the field of manual therapy, spinal mobilisations with arm movement came first but it was not long before I discovered that by using the same principles, the lumbar spine could also be treated when there was a loss of SLR or the patient presented with a positive Femoral Nerve Test. I consider this last technique to be the final chapter in the new field of MWMS as they apply to the vertebral column. As time passes they will however be modified and improved upon. As a therapy they will earn an equal place with other manual therapies currently in use and when you read part two of this book you will be amazed at how extensively they can be applied in the treatment of extremity joints. Back to work!

Firstly let us assume we have a patient with pain laterally in the right lower leg when he straight leg raises to 45 degrees and you suspect a lumbar 4/5 lesion.

There are two starting positions for this MWM , side lying or prone. My choice would be to use the prone position but you may choose the side lying. With the former one assistant is required and with the latter there must be three of you when the patient is in great pain.

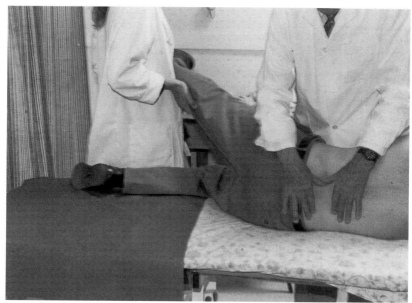

Figure 32a

Spinal mobilisations with leg movement (SMWLMS) with assistant.

Figure 32b

"SMWLMS" showing thumb positioning.

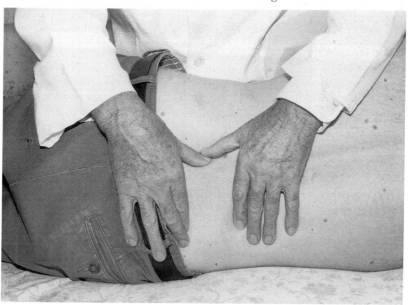

Side lying

Have the patient facing you , lying on his left side with your assistant supporting his right leg (See figure 32a). When a patient is in side lying the upper leg is automatically in hip adduction due to the width of the pelvis. With an acute lumbar lesion ensure that the leg is raised so that the hip is abducted approximately 10'. If you do not do this pain may prevent the patient from lying on his side. You flex over the patient and place one thumb reinforced by the other on the right side of Lumbar 4's spinous process. (See figure 32b) This is often tender to touch so place a piece of plastic foam under your thumb.

Now push down on the chosen spinous process which will side flex the spine at that level and rotate that vertebra on the one below. Sustain this pressure and have the patient actively SLR the supported leg in the side lying position provided there is no pain. As with the previous three techniques repeat three times then test again the straight leg raise when the patient is in a supine position. Satisfaction can almost be guaranteed but do no more than this on day one. On subsequent visits, as the patient improves, your assistant can apply overpressure, again with the understanding that there is no discomfort. The spinous process of lumbar 5 is chosen if the patient has a L5/S1 lesion. I hate to use superlatives, as the reader has probably already noticed, but when this technique works there is no other word for it other than exciting.

Prone lying. (Remember you need two assistants.)

The patient lies prone and slightly obliquely so that he can attempt to straight leg raise the painful leg over the side of the bed. (You require a treatment bed that can be raised to a height to allow the leg to SLR sufficiently). It is essential when they are in position that one assistant takes the weight of the leg. Sometimes the patient is so disabled that pillows, under the abdomen, to flex the lumbar spine in this position are necessary for comfort. A pillow to flex the spine is often a good idea anyway as the spinous processes are more accessible and it allows an even greater range of SLR to take place in the tall patient, when this stage has been reached. Assuming the patient has a Lumbar 4/5 lesion, you now stand on the affected side and place one thumb, reinforced by the other, on the side of Lumbar 4's spinous process. Your second assistant places her thumbs on the side of Lumbar 5's spinous process. Now strongly push the L4 process transversly away from you while your second assistant transversly moves L5 towards you. Sustain, and ask the patient to gently take, his well supported leg, towards the floor as far as he can **without pain.**

He stops as soon as he feels any discomfort and the assistant supporting the leg lifts it up to the starting position. If the patient tries to raise his own leg the accompanying lumbar muscle contraction prevents you from remaining on the spinous processes.

Three repetitions only please, if the patient is responding. On subsequent visits many more can be done and when the patient is feeling much better you can have your assistant apply overpressure to the SLR. At this stage I perhaps would not use an assistant to hold the leg and instead place my leg over the patient's and apply overpressure with it.

Secondly let us assume the patient has a positive femoral nerve sign on the right.

Side lying.

Have the patient facing you on his left side. Your assistant would stand behind the patient supporting the right with the knee flexed to 90'. (See figure 32c) You now choose the spinous process of lumbar 2 or 3 and push it down with your thumbs while the patient extend the hip of his supported leg, provided there is no pain.

Prone lying.

In the prone position the assistant supporting the leg would stand beside you. You would be pushing on say, Lumbar 2 while your other assistant would be on Lumbar 3. **Important** here, is that the leg must be raised cautiously by the therapist supporting it provided there is no pain. The patient must let you know as soon as they feel any discomfort. If the patient tries to raise his own leg the contraction of his lumbar muscles will prevent you from making

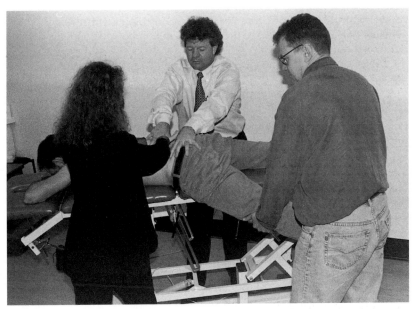

Figure 32c

"SMWLMS" in prone lying with two assistants.

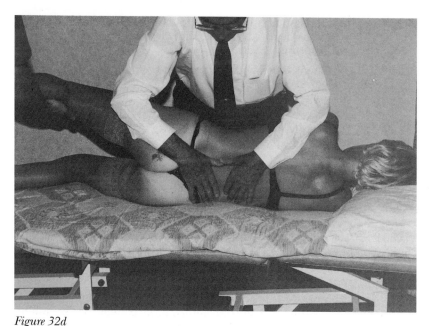

Figure 32d

"SMWLMS" in side lying for positive femoral nerve sign.

contact with the spinous processes. One of our patients this year had lost control of his bladder He had a positive femoral nerve sign and considerable anterior thigh pain.

After five treatments using **SMWLM'S** he was fine. We were all on cloud nine.

H. Sitting

One of the problems encountered when treating the lumbar spine is the difficulty that most patients have with sitting.

Kneeler chairs have proved useful but many cannot tolerate them because of knee complications and the fact that they have no back support. To place a lumbar roll assists in maintaining a lordosis but not a natural one when the hips are flexed beyond 90 degrees to the trunk and the seat back is upright. As soon as your hips are below your knees sitting, as in most cars, you can have a problem. We all know that when a patient sits the pressure within the lower lumbar disc is greater than when standing because of the pelvic tilt. The kneeler chair addresses this problem very nicely by lowering the knees and thus adjusting the pelvic tilt. We suggest that our patients sit on a simple stacking chair (see figure 33) with their legs apart so that they can lower their knees to lower the pressure on the bottom discs and thus form the natural lordosis they have when standing. As you will see from the photograph there is a convenient space for their 'behinds' to fit in when they sit correctly right back in the chair and when positioned correctly the back pad gives appropriate support. The simple chair still posed a problem for ladies in particular as it is not an elegant sitting posture and some patients found that their hips were not flexible enough to straddle the chair.

Now in this edition of the book I must tell you of an easy temporary solution. Take a bed pillow, fold it in half and place it on the back half of the chair and sit on it. Unbelievably effective I hate to say. I get patients to take a pillow to work or the theatre and use it this way. An added bonus at the theatre, if you are short, is that you are now able to see over those inconsiderate tall people sitting in front of you.

I. Spinal Tapings

I use rolls and rolls of 5 cm wide zinc oxide tape in my practice for I tape many spines.

As the upper thoracic spine is readily upset with poor posture and especially with over reaching, taping maintains a good posture and speeds up recovery. With some females I tie their brassiere straps at the back and this often assists.

Many patients experiencing pain with full end range neck rotation will be symptomless if you hold the shoulder girdle back when the movement takes place. If so tape them for a few days.

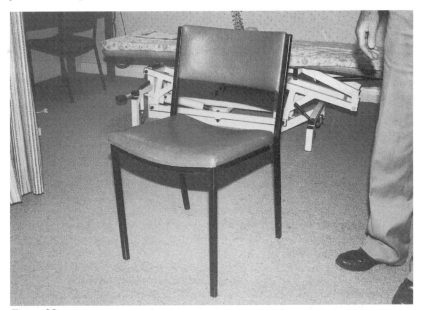

Figure 33
The simple stacking chair.

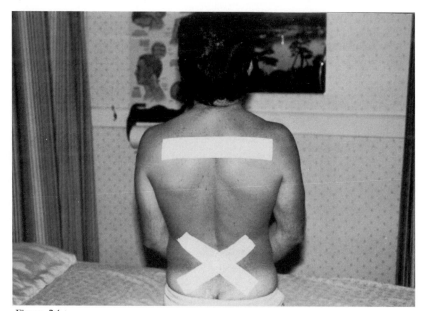

Figure 34

Spinal tapings

With acute lower dorsal and lumbar lesions I tape the patient after 'SNAGS' etc. This reminds them to maintain a good posture and they are grateful for this support. (See figure 34).

J. Exercises

Two exercises are routinely given to all our patients with lumbar lesions provided they produce no pain. One deals primarily with the disc and the other with the facet joints. We tell patients that they ensure a holistic approach which of course is a current buzz word. I believe that dealing with both the facets and the disc in a treatment session has enhanced my treatment outcomes.

1. (For the disc) We get them to do 10 extensions in lying (half press ups a la McKenzie) provided there is no pain at all. We insist that the hands be placed on the bed as close to the waist as possible. This reduces the facet jamming effect when they extend. If they experience unilateral pain we would place a pillow under the hip on that side to see if this removes it. SNAGS with this exercise are extremely useful. With central pain with extension prone, we SNAG them centrally hooking on the spinous process using the radial border of the hand. We would SNAG the appropriate transverse process if it is unilateral using the radial border of the hand. (See figure 35a) When SNAGS eliminate the pain the patient feels much better after 10 repetitions.

My wife Dawn was disabled a couple of years ago with an acute Lumbar 2/3 lesion. She was unable to stand erect had severe pain radiating down her left anterior thigh. Her Femoral nerve test was positive. She could only lie prone when three pillows were placed under her abdomen. I SNAGGED on the transverse process of Lumbar 2 and she was able to do a half press up. After several repetitions she was able to stand erect and the referred pain disappeared. SNAGS in standing completed the cure. How embarrassing it would have been if I had not been able to help her.

2. (For the facets). Following extensions in lying we teach the **'Lion Technique'**. 'Lion exercises' are also given if a patient has been lying prone for any length of time. If extensions in lying could not be undertaken without pain we may only suggest Lion exercises.

They are undertaken with the patient on his hands and knees. This can be done on the bed or floor.

The patient has his knees well apart. Keeping his hands in this starting position he flexes his knees and hips so that his 'behind' moves towards the space provided between his feet. He 'stretches out' his spine in this way , sustains the stretch, rocks forward for a rest and then repeats the stretch 10 times. Because his knees are apart, when viewed from the side, the movement taking place is similar to that with the bent leg raise technique. Patients feel a grand sense of relief when doing this. They can sustain the stretch for a few

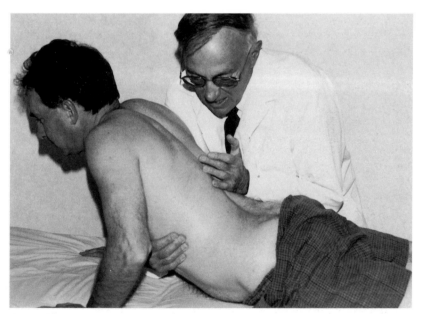

Figure 35a

"SNAGS" with passive extension in lying.

seconds and repeat the exercises many times through the day provided they find that it is useful and of course with the technique they must experience no pain. If they did they would not use it. Even patients with an acute lesion will often find relief from it. We can further improve the technique by placing a pillow under the knee on the affected side. This not only emphasises the BLR on the effected side which is a bonus but introduces a rotation component which can also be a bonus. The rotation introduced is appropriate if the two leg rotation or gate technique had been successful.

Better still! Apply a SNAG centrally to the spinous process or unilaterally over the appropriate transverse process with the radial border of your hand while they do the Lion exercise. Patients love it and the outcome can be spectacular. (Figure 35b)

We always ask patients to do 10 Lion exercises after they have been prone for any length of time and after any prone extensions in lying (half pressups). This frees up the facet joints.

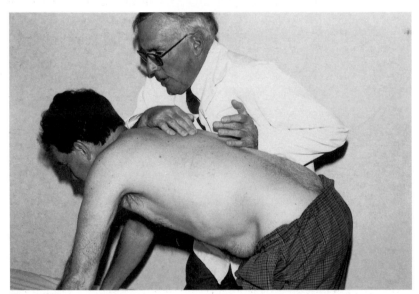

Figure 35b

"SNAGS" with the "Lion" exercises.

PART TWO

THE EXTREMITIES. MOBILISATIONS WITH MOVEMENT. (MWMS)

Explanation

There is nothing new in mobilisation and nothing new in movement to be dealt with in this section. It is the combination of the two modalities that is being advocated. When successful the results that can be obtained are spectacular.

I consider them a breakthrough in the management of extremity joint restrictions and also in dealing with some apparent soft tissue lesions.

Mobilisations with movement (MWMS) will require professional validation to be included in the syllabi of orthodox manual therapy courses. However I predict that this will occur quickly once manipulative therapists become acquainted with and start to use them. To assist in their promotion I am building up a library of video material showing their efficacy on patients in my clinic. When I use these film clips on the lecture circuit they make a substantial impact on colleagues not to mention the patients involved at the time of their treatment.

The reader will observe that I did not specify active movement with mobilisation because there is a place for passive movement and passive overpressure is a key to their success.

In addition there is a place for active contractions of muscles around a joint with mobilisation. The pain experienced with the standard muscle contraction tests for chronic "tennis elbow" will usually disappear when undertaken with an appropriate elbow joint mobilisation.

It would appear to me, the unscientific observer, that this new treatment approach (MWMS) is required for one basic reason.

I consider that minor positional faults occur following injury or strain resulting in movement restrictions and/or pain. These are not readily palpable or visible on x-ray but when a correctional mobilisation (a repositioning) is sustained, pain free function is restored and several repetitions will begin to bring lasting improvements. When a loss of supination in a forearm, for over 30 years, can be restored passively in seconds by repositioning the ulnar in relation to the radius distally then this technique must be known to all physical therapists. It not only tells us something but it is really exciting. I consider that this theory holds because when you just mobilise the joint in the same direction many times without the movement, and then check the active range there is no change.

Another reason that seems to confirm the position hypothesis is that the mobilisation with the movement is nearly always at right angles to the plane of the movement taking place and will only work in ONE direction. Added to this is that when successful in restoring say flexion the same correction will also restore extension if it is lost. This is far different from the mobilisations currently taught, that are all biomechanically based. You mobilise in one direction for one movement loss and then choose another direction for another movement loss. A further point is that when the correct MWM is repeated several times the joint's option to stay on track seems to return.

These positional faults would appear to occur in all extremity joints and this possibility should be considered when assessing all patients with joint problems. I have on film a young (14yrs) dancer who strained her foot and had been unable to plantar flex for three weeks because of pain. We found that a sustained mobilisation of the base of her second metatarsal down on the third enabled pain free plantar flexion. What was more remarkable was the fact that after several repetitions she was then able to plantar flex painlessly without the mobilisation (positional correction). Although some discomfort was present when she returned two days later further MWMS cleared this and she returned to dancing.

The reader will of course agree, when comparing "SNAGS" with "MWMS", that there is very little difference. They both address the problems of movement pain and restriction, they both bring about a change at the time of delivery, they are painless when indicated and of course they are both examples of a sustained mobilisation with movement. The main difference between the spinal techniques and those for the extremities is that with the former the facet mobilisations are normally in the plane of the active movement taking place and with the extremities the sustained mobilisations to correct a positional fault are applied in a different direction to the movement glide taking place.

With many joints the correction can be maintained with taping. This new form of assessment and therapy began for me with a finger but we can now apply it, when indicated, to all peripheral joints.

Descriptions

Examples of how you may apply MWMS to different extremity joints will now be detailed. Sufficient examples will be given to enable the professional to fully understand the principles so that they will quickly be able to ascertain when, how and why they will use them.

1. The fingers. Loss of and/or pain with interphalangeal joint movement.

We all see patients with restricted hinge joints following injury and the fingers are no exception. A typical therapy routine would be some form of heat followed by active exercises and of course manual therapy. The manual therapy used by most would include traction, ventral or dorsal glides and maybe medial or lateral glides. In my decades as a therapist I have rarely been able to achieve instant success with this format. MWMS are so good as a treatment modality with restricted finger movement that I would humbly suggest they should be your first choice of therapy. I extol their supremacy for two reasons. Firstly the glides are painless as is the active movement taking place. Secondly the restricted range of movement is immediately altered. It is paramount to remember that this therapy should be painless and if not discard it. Another point is that if the range of movement does not alter straight away discard the technique. Simple?

The patient is seated and you stabilise the proximal facet of the stiff and often swollen joint with the pads of your right (or left) index finger and thumb. These are placed medially and laterally. Now secure the distal facet of the joint medially and laterally with your other thumb and index finger. (See figure 36). The distal facet is now glided medially and then laterally. In nearly every case you will find that one direction is painful and the other is not. You choose the direction that is painless and then ask the patient to flex his stiff finger while you sustain the mobilisation. This active movement should be pain free and the range should increase. To complete the MWM have the patient apply some overpressure with his free hand. The overpressure is like the cream on the milk. It enhances the result. This procedure would be repeated several times and the range of movement reassessed.

When we talk about a medial or lateral glide it should be added that the application requires some sensitivity. Remember it must be parallel with the treatment plane. A pain being experienced with a particular glide will often disappear by minimally altering the direction. When you get an instant im-

Figure 36

MWM for loss of interphalangeal joint flexion or extension.

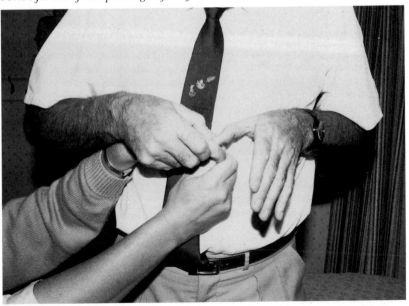

provement in a range of movement with a sustained glide in one direction only, which is at right angles to the glide taking place, what other explanation could there be for its success other than the correction of a positional fault?

In past years I have had a few patients who have not responded to a medial or lateral glide with movement but to a rotation of the distal facet with movement. The first patient was memorable. She was unable to flex the metacarpo/phalangeal of her thumb following a hyperextension injury. Full of confidence I said to her that she would be able to move the joint immediately and without pain when I placed the bone ends in the correct position. To my surprise and well hidden embarrassment I found that neither a medial or a lateral glide made any difference. However because of my conversion to the positional fault belief I tried a medial rotation of the distal facet on the proximal but this was painful. I then rotated the facet in the opposite direction. Brilliant! No pain and she was able to again move her joint. The other three who failed to respond to the glide at right angles also responded to the appropriate rotation. (Aristotle said that you can trust your judgement if it is based on logic?)

When teaching I now tell participants that with mobile hinge joints, excluding the ankle, the appropriate mobilisation to use with movement is usually at right angles to the glide taking place and if these are painful try a rotation. Sometimes a combination lateral glide with a rotation is the magic formula.

With fingers the technique is so simple that patients can be taught to do their own MWMS several times a day. As already mentioned you can expect, when these techniques are indicated and applied, to find that the patient has retained most of the improvement gained at his next treatment session.

2. The metacarpals. Pain when the hand is clenched along say the 5th metacarpal.

There are no joints between adjacent metacarpals. However be on the alert for postitional faults between all adjacent long bones in the body. An excellent example that I must share with you was of a women who three months after a fracture of her fifth metacarpal had pain whenever she gripped anything. The pain was over the proximal third of the bone and she experienced a lot of pain gripping the steering wheel of her car. We found that when the base of the fifth metacarpal was lifted up in relation to the fourth her grip was pain free. Three sets of ten ,of these MWM'S, resulted in pain free gripping without the correction.

She returned two days later feeling much better and only required four treatments. I should add that I taped the base of the fifth metacarpal up on the fourth before she left my rooms to ensure that the bone remained in 'the corrected position'.

3. The carpal bones

Mobilisations with movement have proved to be the solution with many patients with localised functional pain in the carpus. An example would be a patient who experiences pain over the dorsal aspect of his trapezium with gripping. In my teaching video a patient is presented with such a problem of 9 months' duration, after a crush injury. Specialists were unable to offer an explanation for his misery. We found that by 'repositioning' his trapezium ventrally in relation to the scaphoid he could clench his fist with no discomfort. I must admit that it took several attempts to get the right direction of the glide so that there was no discomfort. As with the earlier MWMS we would have him gripping strongly 10 times with the sustained mobilisation. After three sets he would depart almost pain free and after six treatments was discharged.

On my courses I now teach that with joints in the body that only have small ranges of movement, the mobilisation with movement is really to reposition one facet up or down on its neighbour with movement as an assessment to see if it is indicated. On my courses, in the US alone, we have seen dozens of therapists with pain over their scaphoids with wrist extension. They are unable to weight bear on their extended wrists. (Like a press up). Reposition the scaphoid up or down on the lower end of the radius and you will find that the movement is now pain free. Repetitions with over pressure bring about a resolution. I have hundreds of witnesses to confirm how effective these procedures can be. The other point that I make after dealing with the fingers, metacarpals and carpus, is that on the basis of the MWMS for these joints you now have guidelines to assess and treat when indicated all the joints of the body.

As you read on you will see how pertinent this comments is.

4. The wrist joint. A loss of and pain with flexion and/or extension.

As with the fingers the accompanying mobilisation with the movement is usually a medial or lateral glide. With the wrist I have found that the successful glide has been a lateral one and I would like to describe this first of all.

The patient is seated. You stand proximal to and grasp the lower ends of the radius and ulna with one hand so that the web between your index finger and thumb lies over the distal end of the radius. The web between the thumb and index finger of your other hand lies medially over the proximal row of carpal bones keeping the rest of your fingers and thumb from making contact with the patient. (See figure 37a). You now glide the carpals laterally. If this is painful, ever so slightly, alter the direction of the glide to seek a pain free glide. Provided this can be achieved , maintain the mobilisation and have the patient actively move in the restricted direction. (Flexion or extension). If the MWM is indicated the range of movement will improve instantly and of course painlessly. Repeat ten times always having the patient apply overpressure with his free hand to get further range. After three sets of ten the patient should now find that they can move, without positional correction, much more freely.

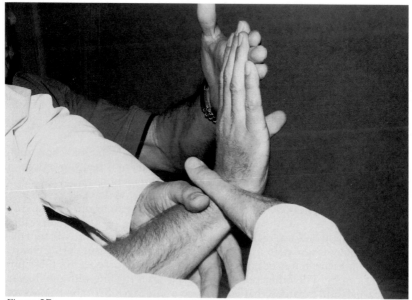

Figure 37a

MWM for wrist flexion or extension.

Figure 37b

Taping to maintain lateral glide of carpals.

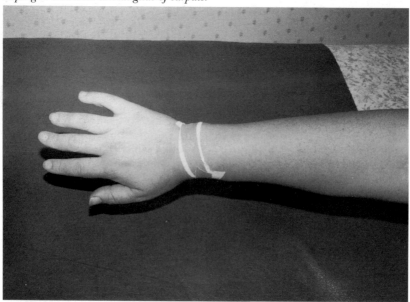

A useful adjunct to a successful MWM is to apply tape diagonally across the wrist joint to maintain the useful glide.(See figure 37b).

It may interest the reader to know that we recently treated a 35 year old woman who presented with a dorsal wrist ganglion as well as pain and a loss of wrist flexion. The ganglion and painful movement loss followed a jarring injury three weeks earlier. With our first sustained lateral glide she was able to fully flex her wrist painlessly and the ganglion immediately reduced in size. After six repetitions she had full pain free function and the swelling had dissipated. We were fortunate enough to record her treatment at the time on video tape.

If a lateral glide is not successful in allowing pain free movement you rotate the proximal row of carpals on the radius and ulna to see if this repositioning allows the wrist to function. As to whether you rotate medially or laterally is for you to find out. The reader will now see that the approach is no different to that taken with a finger. The rotation can be sustained with taping and we found this taping extremely effective in removing pain and swelling from the osteoarthritic wrist of a 65 year old woman.

Finally you may have to combine a rotation with a glide for success as the wrist is a complex structure.

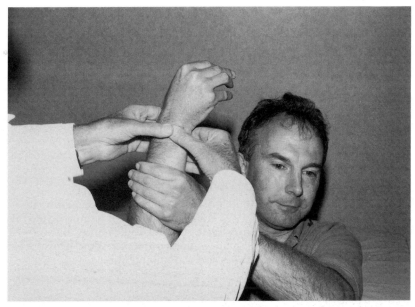

Figure 38

MWM for forearm supination loss.

5. The distal radio-ulnar joint. Pain and/or movement loss with supination and/or pronation.

With this joint an altered relationship between the distal ends of the radius an ulna can cause pain and movement loss. If dealing with a right wrist this would be the routine.

For a loss of supination

With the patient sitting, stand proximal to the right wrist. Place the fingers of your left hand anteriorly along the ulnar border of the radius for an accurate stablisation. Place you right thumb over the lower end of the ulna. Now put your left thumb over the right one and push the ulnar down on the radius . The fingers of your right hand would lie over those of your left. With the ulna now repositioned on the radius have the patient supinate with overpressure provided there is no pain. Make sure your hands go with the movement. You will get amazing results using this technique after Colles' fractures and even long standing restrictions. (See figure 38). If this were painful move the radius dorsally on the ulna.

For a loss of pronation

The procedure is the same as above but stand distal to the joint and it is much easier.

In the old days I would try and restore movement in the forearm by mobilising in the biomechanically correct direction and then reassess movement. I do not recall anything spectacular ever happening. Supporting the positional fault hypothesis is the fact the repositioning that restores say supination will also restore pronation. If the MWM is indicated then no pain will be experienced with movement and several repetitions will make a tremendous difference. It would then be easy to tape the ulna in its corrected position if you thought it desirable. Using this technique on one of my courses in America a therapist with a 32 year loss of supination regained full movement in one session before 70+ colleagues. It made quite an impact.

6. The elbow joint. Movement losses and Tennis Elbow.

Basically the elbow is a hinge joint and this prompted me to experiment with the above conditions to see if MWMS might apply in their treatment and they most certainly do. In 1990 I succeeded in dramatically improving an 8 year loss of flexion in a 44 year old man in one treatment session. This was certainly exceptional and I have video corroboration of this.

a. Movement losses.

The patient is lying on his back with his arm on the plinth and forearm supinated. You wrap the now familiar belt around your hips and his forearm so that the proximal edge is level with the elbow joint. You stabilise the lower end of his humerus with one hand and support the forearm with the other. The stabilising hand and forearm lie within the belt. Your elbow should rest in the flexor crease of your hip. (See figure 39a). You now glide the ulna laterally with the belt by moving you hips gently away. Little force is used. Provided there is no pain the patient then actively bends or extends his elbow while you maintain the mobilisation. You can add a little overpressure with your distally placed hand. If the patient is extending, remember that with the carrying angle at the elbow, the treatment plane alters slightly with the movement and you must alter the direction of your glide to deal with this. Depending on your size and that of the patient's elbow you may choose not to use a belt. Instead you can secure the lower end of the humerus with one hand and apply the glide with your other hand. To do this position the lateral border of the 2nd metacarpo/phalangeal joint of your free hand over the upper end of the ulna at the joint margin. (See figure 39b).

The reader will note from the photograph that I make no skin contact with the rest of my mobilising hand. I do not want it to block movement. When both hands are busy in this way I get the patient to apply passive overpressure to the movement.

As with all the other MWMS already dealt with in this book remember that other forms of therapy would be given as well. No pain!

If the glides are not successful we have found that sometimes there is a radial head positional fault. This may be palpable. When suspected push the radial head forward on the humerus and sustain while the patient tries to flex or extend (with overpressure and without pain). Other directions for the radial head should also be considered.

b. Tennis elbow.

With long standing tennis elbows (over three weeks) we have been using a new routine involving MWMS and have had some interesting successes.

The treatment is to make the patient exercise his forearm repeatedly in any way that is (on testing) painful but . . . the exercise is done with a sustained mobilisation and must be painless. (See figure 40a). Let us assume that the patient is unable, when the elbow is extended and the forearm pronated, to clench his fist without pain. We have found that in nearly every case, when a lateral glide is applied at the elbow joint, the patient experiences no pain with gripping. When this has been repeated 10 times he should then be able to clench the fist with less discomfort without the concurrent mobilisation. Interesting? On early visits three sets of 10 or more may be needed to rid all of the symptoms when gripping. The only problem after several sets of the above is that the patient will have difficulty bending his elbow. To correct this do 6 repetitions of the above with the elbow flexed at 30' then 60' and finally 90'. Be it painful wrist or finger extension or gripping pain the same lateral glide seems to work. Sometimes it takes three or four attempts to get the gliding direction exactly right but when on target it's great. We usually, as an assessment, use our hands in the manner described for elbow restrictions rather than the belt to ascertain if the MWM will be of value. For these MWMS to work, with what is thought to be a soft tissue lesion, there must be a tracking or positional fault at the elbow contributing in no small way to chronic tennis elbow.

We still use tennis elbow bracing and other therapy at the same time. The patients are instructed to exercise regularly at home. They are shown how to self mobilise so that the exercises are pain free. If they cannot successfully self mobilise then the exercises are not given.

One way of self gliding the extended elbow is to use a doorway. Stand with the upper arm against the wall so that the elbow joint is level with the opening. Now push the ulna laterally using the web space between the index finger and thumb of the free hand. (See figure 40b). After a few sets of self MWMS the patient should be able to exercise without pain.

Sometimes with tennis elbow the grip is painful through a range of elbow flexion so the MWMS would be undertaken with altered elbow flexion. A variation to the lateral glide with movement has been required with some tennis elbows when pain has been produced with gripping when the elbow was at a right angle. When the flexed elbow was distracted with a belt the pain with gripping was eliminated. (See figure 40c).

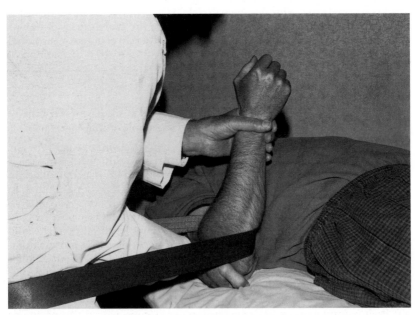

Figure 39a

MWM for movement loss at elbow using belt.

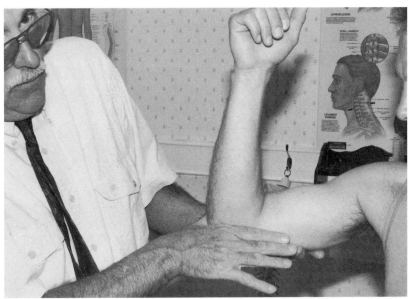

Figure 39b

MWM for elbow movement loss using hands.

Figure 40a

MWM for tennis elbow using belt in lying.

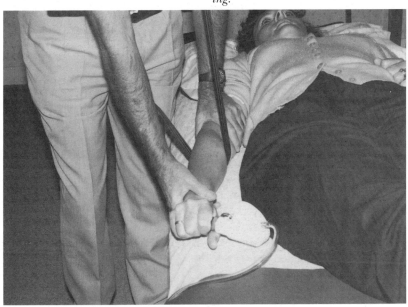

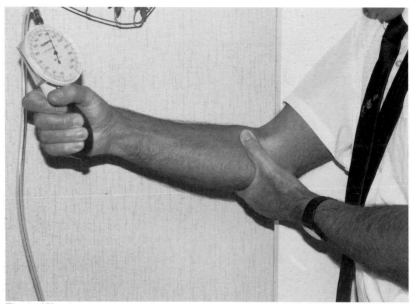

Figure 40b

Self MWM for tennis elbow using doorway.

Figure 40c

MWM. Distraction with movement at elbow using belt.

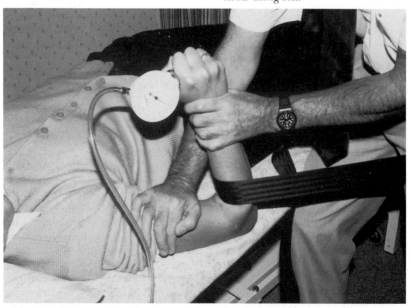

Manual Therapy

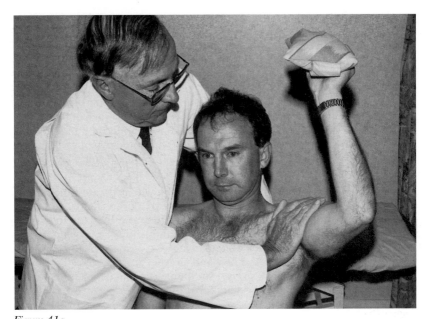

Figure 41a

MWM for shoulder elevation through abduction.

While on the subject of Tennis Elbow could I refer the reader back to the section on Cervical Mobilisations with Arm Movements. If MWMS do not work or there are still residual symptoms after their use try moving Cervical 4 (or 5) across away from the affected side and re test for tennis elbow. Worth a try and I will say no more.

7. The shoulder joint. Painful movement losses, rotator cuff lesions etc.

The applications of MWMS for shoulder joint lesions can be rewarding. They certainly have a place and in this new edition I wish to deal with some of the uses for them.

Let us consider the application of MWMS to a right shoulder that is painful when raised above 90 degrees through abduction (typical with a rotator cuff lesion). The patient is seated. You stand at his left side with your right hand over his left scapula and the thenar eminence of your left hand over the head of the humerus. You ask the patient to raise his arm up from his side while you apply a postero/lateral gliding force over the head of the humerus with your left hand. (You avoid pressure over the sensitive corocoid process by being just below and medial to it). (See figure 41a) When indicated and you are correctly positioned the arm will rise painlessly. As with the finger, wrist and elbow, the mobilisation that seems to work is at right angles to the active glide taking place. Is it a positional fault that inhibits pain free movement? If the technique is successful the next step is to have the patient, while you retain the repositioning, 'punch' his arm up to full flexion ten times under load by giving them a weight to lift as in the Figure 41a. Three sets or more of ten should result in much better shoulder function. This MWM (with a weight) would be used on each visit with other modalities until the lesion has recovered. You will note that I said to push the head of the humerus posteriorly. We have never had any success with an anterior glide but this possibility should not be excluded. As with the MWMS for the other joints, after several repetitions, patients should notice a marked improvement and much of this should be retained between visits. Many quickly learn how to apply their own MWMS. This technique has proved instantly successful with some patients who have a gross loss of movement, usually with some swelling, following a fall on or a blow to the shoulder.

To dorsally glide the humerus of a large patient, when you are small in stature, is simple when you use a belt. (See figure 41b) You stand behind the seated patient and place the belt around your hips and the patient's shoulder. Place a hand on the scapular for fixation and lean back in such a way as to glide the humeral head back obliquely in the treatment plane. Your free hand's fingers would secure the belt and prevent it from slipping. Ensure that the belt does not slightly elevate the humeral head as this will jam the joint and inhibit movement. Remember no pain and the usual repetitions etc.

Figure 41b

MWM with belt for shoulder abduction.

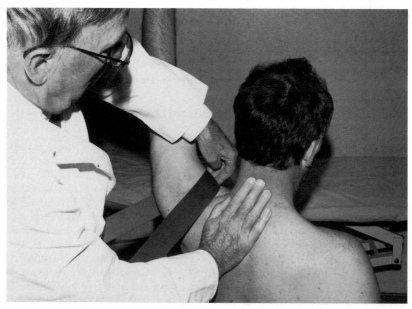

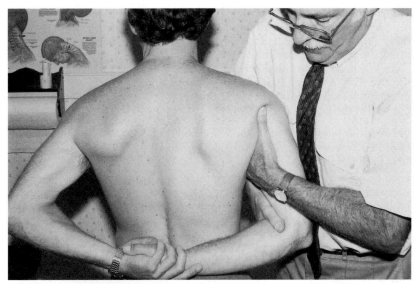

Figure 42a

MWM *for internal rotation.*

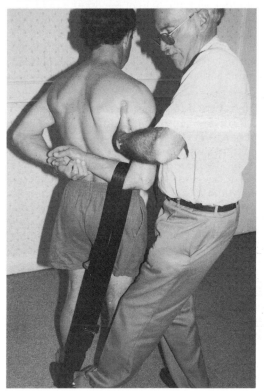

Figure 42b

MWM *for internal rotation using belt.*

There is now another way of doing this. Lie the patient supine and at the head of the bed grasp the humerus with one hand and the forearm with the other on the effected side. Now push down along the shaft of the humerus while the patient tries to raise his arm. This procedure does two things. It glides the head of the humerus dorsally on the glenoid and also down when the arm is above 90' which is a bonus. In endeavouring to achieve an increase in flexion look for a pain free direction. Move the arm up further away from the side of the head.

Another movement loss that can respond spectacularly to a MWM is **internal rotation** provided the patient can get his thumb around as far as his sacrum. (See figure 42 a).

For a loss of right internal rotation, stand facing the patient's right side. Place your right thumb in the bend of his flexed right elbow. His hand should be as far behind his back as possible. Now place the web between your finger and thumb in the patient's axilla. You now glide the head of the humerus down in the glenoid fossa using your right thumb while stabilising the scapula with your left hand. Make sure the your left hand is stabilising up and inwards. If not you will place a pressure on the upper end of the humerus which is both unpleasant and ineffective. While this distraction is taking place have the patient internally rotate his shoulder, with the help of the other hand if necessary, while you adduct his upper arm using your abdomen. As you push into adduction in this way the head of the humerus is distracted laterally. The hand in the axilla acts as a fulcrum. It all sounds very complex but it is not difficult to do and patients amazingly tolerate the technique and experience no pain. What is more important is that in most cases internal rotation is increased.

There is an alternative way of doing this using your treatment belt instead of your thumb.(See figure 42b) Place the belt in the bend of the elbow and have the loop about 6 centimetres from the floor when it lies obliquely behind the patient's back. For the right shoulder, place your left forefoot in the loop ensuring that your heel is on the floor. As the belt lies obliquely, when pressure is applied in the bend of the elbow as your foot plantarflexes, the emphasis is where your thumb would have been. That is right on the joint margin which does not prevent the forearm from flexing up behind the back. Your two overlapping hands are placed in the axilla to stabilise the scapula and they thus act as a greater fulcrum when you use your abdomen to adduct the arm behind the patient's back.

8. The acromio-clavicular and sterno clavicular joints.

A Therapist on one of my courses had not been able to elevate her arm beyond 140' for 15 years. Shoulder MWMS made no difference . I then repositioned her acromio-clavicular joint by pushing firmly down and back on the outer end of the clavicle and asked her to raise her arm. She regained full shoulder movement before 70+ disbelieving colleagues. Three months later she still had full function. What about adaptive shortening??

Similarly if you suspect the sterno-clavicular, reposition the proximal end of the clavicle down and back and have the patient undertake the shoulder movement involved.

9. The foot

Foot injuries abound due to the participation in impact sporting activities by an increasing percentage of the public at large over recent years. Never before have the streets of our cities been so overwhelmed with runners and there has been a proliferation of fitness centres crammed with devotees.

The foot should be treated in the same way as the hand . Toes respond like fingers, the metatarsals like the metacarpals and positional faults should be considered when pain is experienced with movement of the tarsals.

To introduce you to the application of mobilisations with movement as a foot therapy I will deal with two areas where pain with movement can be experienced. However, when foot movement causes localised foot pain a 'MWM' should always be tried. It can quickly be established if it is indicated as it would allow the offending movement to take place painlessly.

a. Pain over the medial border of the foot with inversion.

This can be due to a 'positional' fault at the base of the first metatarsal. The patient's foot is on a plinth. You stand beside and proximal to the foot to be treated. (Let us assume a left one). You place the ventral shaft of the first

Figure 43

MWM First metatarsal base on second with inversion.

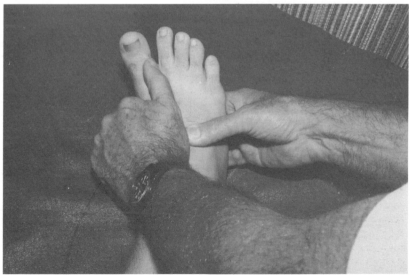

metacarpal of your right hand along the dorsum of the shaft of the patient's first metatarsal. The fingers of this hand lie firmly beneath this metatarsal so the bone is secured. The fingers of your left hand lie under the foot along the shaft of the second metatarsal and the thumb on top.(See figure 43). Now glide the base of the first metatarsal down on the second and while maintaining this ask the patient to invert the foot provided there is no pain. Your fingers beneath the second metatarsal apply a counter pressure up on the second metatarsal. If the inversion is now pain free have the patient repeat the movement with mobilisation many times. (Ten?). When successful they will now have painless active inversion without mobilisation. To assist your therapy a positional taping can be used for a few days.

Although it is usually a ventral glide that works it may be the other direction that is required so you alter your hand placements for the MWMS.

Sometimes the base of the first metatarsal needs to be positioned dorsally or ventrally on the first cunneiform, or the cuneiform on the navicular or the base of the fifth metatarsal on the cuboid. Experience and experimentation unite when feet are being treated with this approach.

b. Anterior metatarsalgia. Pain under the transverse arch.

If pain under the heads of the middle metatarsals can be reproduced with toe flexion or extension this could be due to a metatarsal head positional fault and a MWM should be tried.

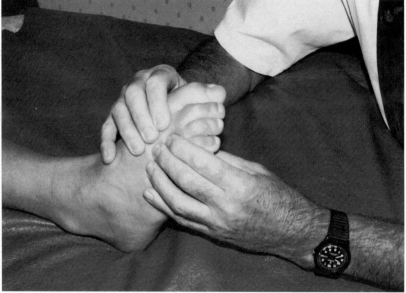

Figure 44

MWM for anterior metatarsalgia. See text.

With the patient's foot on the plinth stand distally and grasp the head of say the third metatarsal between the soft pads of your thumb and index finger. Your other thumb and index finger grasps the head of the adjacent second. Now glide and hold the third down on the second while the patient flexes his toes. (See figure 44). If painful, glide the second down on the third.

When painless repeat six to ten times and then have the patient flex his toes without assistance to reassess. After several sets he should feel much better. We would follow this therapy with corrective exercises and perhaps appropriate taping.

10. The Ankle Joint

The ankle joint is a delight to treat when there is a loss of plantar or dorsiflexion and the technique I will describe for the former I call the 100% miracle technique. The technique for dorsiflexion I call the 97% miracle technique. Both of course are MWMS but the former was in fact shown to me by Professor F M Kaltenborn in 1974. It was not taught as an MWM of course and sadly the significance of the procedure escaped me (and others) for many years.

a. Plantar flexion loss.

Let us assume that your patient has a loss of movement in his right ankle. He

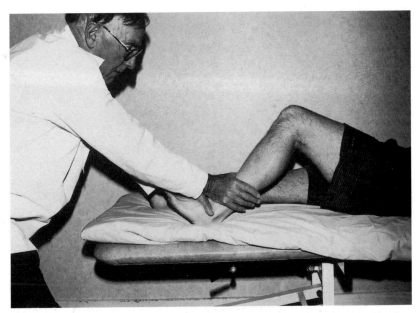

Figure 45
"Miracle" MWM for plantar flexion.

reclines on a couch with his right knee and heel flexed to 90' and the heel is on the bed. You stand at the end facing him. Place the hypothenar border of your left hand just proximal to the joint line and wrap your thumb and fingers insecurely around the lower leg. (See figure 45) Pressure will be delivered evenly on both the tibia and fibula with the hypothenar aspect of the hand.

Now place the webbing between the thumb and index finger of your right hand around the talus. Your thumb and index fingers would slope slightly distally so that they lie just below the malleolae. Stand in a lunge position with your left elbow wedged in your left groin. Using your body weight glide the tibia and fibula posteriorly as far as you can. This locks the ankle joint. Without releasing this glide roll the talus ventrally with your right hand provided no pain is produced. If it were, the good therapist would slightly alter the direction to see if this eliminates the pain. Very little movement is expected due to the slack being taken up in the joint by your left arm. What movement you do get is in fact restored plantar flexion. Several repetitions ensure a marked and lasting improvement.

Patients would exercise to maintain the range.

Forgive the tedious reminders but this MWM must not hurt. Often after fractures the tissues around the ankle are swollen and thus tender. As on other occasions use some plastic foam under your hands for patient comfort.

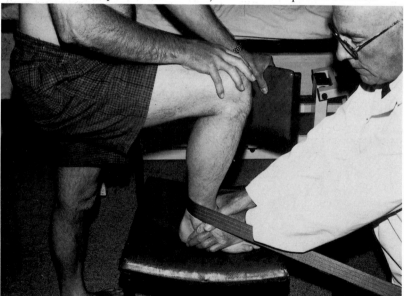

Figure 46

MWM for dorsiflexion.

b. Dorsiflexion loss.

Let us assume that your patient has a loss of movement in his right ankle.

Have the patient standing with his right foot on a chair. Place the ever useful belt around your hips and the patient's lower leg about 4cms above the insertion of the tendo-achilles. Between the belt and the tendo achilles you must place a folded towel for comfort. (See figure 46) Now wrap the web between the thumb and index finger of one hand, reinforced by the other around the talus as close to the joint margin as possible. Pull the tibia and fibula forward with the belt as the patient, holding the back of the chair, flexes forward over his foot. As usual there must be no pain; if there was have the patient alter slightly the direction that the knee takes over the fixated foot. Subtle directional changes are often the keys to success. The good manual therapist would be alert to this . When the patient comes forward the lower leg slopes towards you so you must lower your hips to maintain a good contact with the belt. I used to teach a non weight bearing MWM for this joint but no longer do so. The reason is that when movement is gained in weight bearing it is kept. When gained non weight bearing it is often lost when the patient stands up. At the same time the patient actively forces further dosiflexion by flexing his knee. Several repetitions please and reassess.

11. a. The distal tibio/fibular joints and inversion sprains of the ankle.

In dealing with this joint I would like to suggest that all practitioners in the medical and allied medical fields have been so so wrong in the diagnosis of many ankle strains. I believe and also hope to convince you that almost every patient diagnosed as having strained the talo-fibular ligament of the ankle has not, or if some fibres have been torn the damage is of little significance. The problem resulting from inversion strains lies within the distal tibio/fibular joint. I believe that when the foot is forcibly inverted beyond the natural range the lateral ligament usually remains undamaged. The fibula gets wrenched forward on the tibia and positional faults occur. In fact the ligament is so strong that often the tip of the lateral maleollus fractures. It surprises me that this joint has not been the focus of attention with ankle sprains. Many text books tell us that with severe ankle sprains the superior tibio-fibular joint is involved; with this being the case we should have concentrated more on the distal joint.

To describe the technique let me do so with a case history. In 1992 a middle aged man limped in to see me 6 weeks after he 'went over' on his ankle. His foot was swollen and he had no inversion at all. On assessment I found that when I glided his fibula back on his tibia and held it there he was able to fully invert his foot with NO PAIN. After the usual MWM repetitions I taped his fibula dorsally on his tibia and he left my rooms feeling 90% better. On his return two days later most of his swelling had gone and he had only minimal discomfort at the end of full range inversion. MWMS were again used and no further therapy was required. A gratifying result and to me and the only explanation that my simple mind could accept is that he had a positional fault.

Ever since, with all 'lateral ligament' strains of the ankle we have checked the fibula, and I am confident that ankle strains rarely damage the lateral ligament. Most strains involve the tibio/fibular joint. Referring back to the man above I wish to make the following points. Firstly after 6 weeks if the only damage to his ankle was to the lateral ligament why had it not shown any signs of recovery. The swelling could be explained but not the gross loss of inversion. Secondly when the foot is inverted while you are gliding the fibula dorsally the stretch on the lateral ligament is increased. Why did he feel no pain and why was he now able to fully invert his foot painlessly? My explanation, and it is hard to refute it, is that gliding the fibula on the tibia returned the bone to its correct position allowing pain free function to occur. In England in 1994 a therapist on one of my courses had ankle pains and had been unable to invert her foot for 13 years. The fibula was glided dorsally and while this positioning was maintained she was able to get a full active range of inversion. Course participants almost in unison when they saw this mini 'miracle' said 'what about adaptive shortening?' I did not answer their question but the result would have left a lasting impact on all of them. (It was suggested that I might like to go for a walk on the Lake afterwards). (Study figure 47a).

When you glide the fibula, as a test or treatment , do so more or less along the line of the ligament. That is in a dorso cranial direction. Use your thenar eminence and curl your free fingers around the tendo achilles. The thenar eminence of your other hand would lie under the medial malleolus. Ensure you are distally on the malleolus. Your thenar eminence must not be in contact with the ankle joint. This technique will halve the recovery time, reduce your income but give immense satisfaction. When pain is experienced just minimally alter the direction of the movement. You might not have the direction right.

This repositioning of the fibula should be undertaken as soon as possible after an inversion sprain if there is no fracture. In the first 48 hours the RICE protocols are adhered to but with the addition of a taping to hold the fibula 'in place'.

The taping can be seen in figure 47b and is left on for 48 hours provided there is no skin irritation. It lies across the lower leg obliquely, travelling around and up. I use 5cm wide tape. **What should never be done is to tape the foot in eversion as the text books suggest**. This inhibits normal ankle movement and will slow down the healing process. It is pointless! I predict that it will take ten years to get the message all around the world . (2009?)

After 48 hours the MWM routine is used. Glide the fibula dorso-cranially and have the patient do sets of inversion exercises with some overpressure .

We have also repositioned the fibula dorsally with tape to see if this assists in the management of 'shin splints' and at times have been rewarded.

When confronted with a patient with a chronic loss of dorsi flexion ask if he has ever severely sprained his ankle. If he has, reposition the fibula as above while he has his foot on a chair. Now get him to lean forward over his foot to

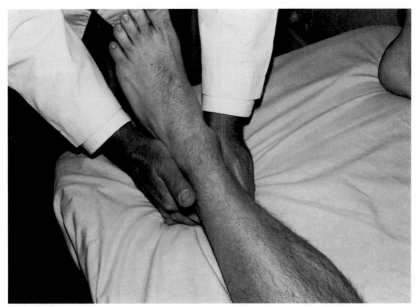

Figure 47a

MWM following inversion ankle strain involving tibio-fibular joint.

Figure 47b

Correct taping for inversion ankle strains.

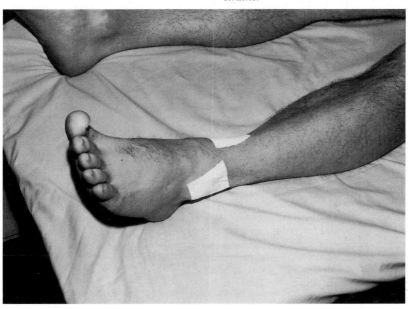

force dorsiflexion. You will probably get an immediate increase in his range of movement.

The MWM following eversion sprains is usually the opposite to the above. Position the fibula ventrally on the tibia while the patient is in prone lying.

Remember overpressure should be used.

b. The proximal tibio/fibular joint.

Be on the lookout for 'positional faults' when postero/lateral knee pain is being experienced. Maybe it is not a biceps tendon strain or a tensor fascia lata syndrome. Take for example the patient who experiences pain in this area with weightbearing knee flexion. Have your patient do this while you are gliding the fibular head forward on the tibia. A good way to achieve this is to have the patient place his foot on a chair and then flex forward over it. (See figure 48). If pain free, do three sets of ten MWMS and reassess. When successful the patient may be able to bend over and SELF MWM using his thenar eminence to glide the fibular head forward. Taping is extremely useful for keeping the fibula head 'in position'.

Patients with the remnants of sciatica down the lateral border of the lower leg to the foot will often experience no pain when the fibula is positioned in this way. This may be because it alters the tension on the nerve responsible.

You will note that my descriptions for MWMS are becoming briefer but it would be tedious to the reader if this were not so. Getting to this stage in the book and with the guidelines mentioned for the fingers, metacarpals and carpus earlier in this section you will probably be orchestrating your own MWMS as different joints are dealt with. This was how I have had to work my way through the joints.

12. The knee joint

MWMS should always be tried when there is a loss of movement that is obviously not the result of serious trauma.

There are two techniques that I will deal with. The first is the medial or lateral glide MWM. The second as expected is the rotation MWM and I would suggest that you read this portion many times because you will find rotation positioning extremely valuable.

The general rule for the gliding direction that I use with movement is 'medial glide with medial knee pain and lateral glide with lateral knee pain'. MWMS are much more likely to assist with a flexion loss than extension. A flexion loss is usually the result of a sporting injury and is often seen when the patient is referred with the diagnosis, collateral ligament strain.

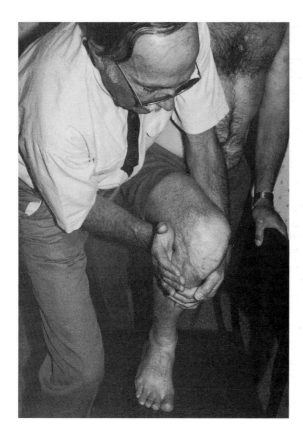

Figure 48

The proximal tibio-fibular joint MWM with weightbearing knee flexion.

The gliding MWM

The patient lies prone and to apply a medial glide you stand on the contralateral side. Place a belt around your waist and the patient's lower leg so that the proximal edge is at the tibial joint margin. To do this you would of course expect the patient to have a reasonable degree of knee flexion. You stabilise the thigh above the knee with one hand and support the lower leg with the other. (See figure 49a). You glide the knee medially with the belt and ask the patient to flex his knee. When indicated the range of movement will immediately improve painlessly. To apply a lateral glide stand beside the restricted knee and use the belt to apply the glide as you did from the other side.

Alternative technique.

I have already generalised in stating that with hinge joints the mobilisation used with movement is usually a medial or lateral glide. However in young adults, particularly sports' persons, who have lost full flexion after leg inju-

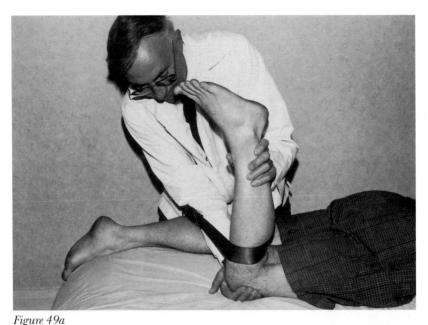

Figure 49a

MWM Medial glide with knee flexion.

ries requiring prolonged immobilisation there is another MWM that can be extremely useful. With this technique the tibial plateau is glided posteriorly (N.B. the treatment plane) first and then the patient flexes his knee while the glide is sustained. It is necessary to have a starting position of at least 80 degrees of flexion before this procedure can be tried.

The patient is supine and you stand beside the knee to be treated. With your fingers interlaced place your hands over the flexed knee so that the heel of one hand lies over the tibial plateau, and the heel of the other is over the lower end of the femur. (See figure 49b). You can now successfully glide the upper end of the tibia posteriorly when you try to proximate the heels of your hands. It is amazing how powerful this technique is so take some care. If you are not right on the upper end of the tibia, or your direction is slightly out, it can be very painful. The patient's contribution here is very important. We usually attach a belt to the ankle of the patient on the restricted side and have her hold this with her hands. When you glide the tibia the patient then actively tries to flex her knee and gets some overpressure by cautiously pulling on the belt. The new position is held for a few seconds and after a short spell the MWM is repeated several times. When indicated the range should increase with each MWM even though it is only a few degrees. It should produce strain and discomfort but not pain. Strong young adults are ideal subjects for this technique but I would not use it on older or very young patients because of the force that can be applied so effortlessly.

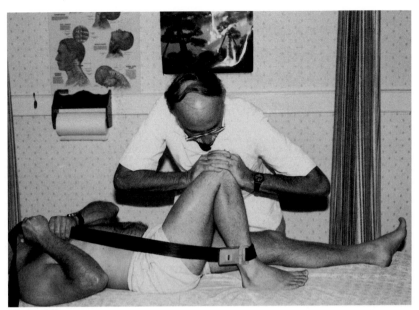

Figure 49b

MWM. Dorsal glide with active knee flexion.

Figure 49c

MWM Rotation supine with knee flexion.

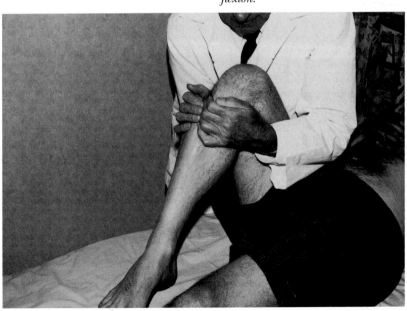

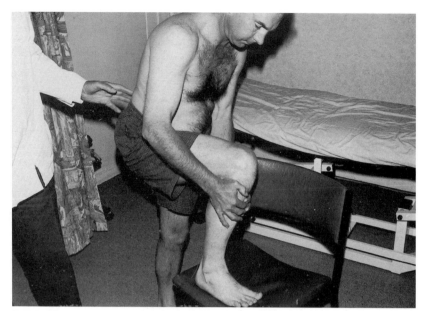

Figure 49d

Self rotation MWMS for flexion on chair.

Rotation MWMS. (These are brilliant even if I say so myself)

If a patient has limited painful knee flexion have the patient supine. Flex up the knee just short of the painful limitation. Now grasp the lower leg and internally rotate the tibia on the femur. It is even better if the fibula is moved ventrally at the same time. (See figure 49c) Maintain this and have the patient flex. When indicated they will be able to flex further without pain. You can apply the overpressure through your hands.

A patient can do his own rotation MWMS with the painful leg on a chair. He places his hands proximally around the lower leg and rotates his tibia medially. (See figure 49d) If the hand on the fibular side carries this forward at the same time it is a bonus. Sustaining this rotation he now bends forward to flex his knee (weightbearing) provided there is no pain. I have my patients with OA knees do this on a regular basis as a home treatment. When rotation is successful, tape the tibia in internal rotation on the femur. The way that I will describe this was suggested to me on one of my courses by an quick thinking colleague, Susan Phillips in Portland, Maine. I liked her way because it is just as effective as the way that I would do it but, with Sue's way, the patient can do it themselves.

The patient stands with his knee flexed about 5-10'. He inverts his foot as far as he can on the femur. 5cm tape is now wrapped diagonally so that the upper edge crosses just below the joint margin. Half the tape would be on the

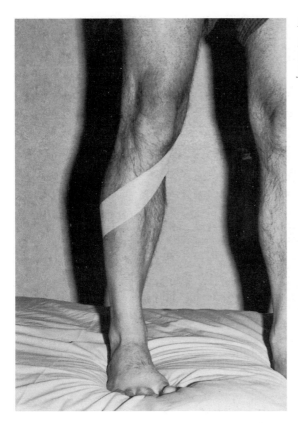

Figure 49e
Knee taping to maintain internal rotation (Wonderful!).

lower leg laterally and the other half wrap around the thigh medially. (See figure 49e)

The number of knee conditions that feel better with this taping is incredible. One unexpected bonus is when the patient has patella femoral problems. Internally rotating the tibia in this way alters the tracking of the patella. Patients who have not responded to the conventional McConnail taping will usually be fine with this.

TAPE - SKIN REACTIONS

I should mention that on one of my February, 1998, courses in the US, therapists told me that they were using "Mylanta" antacid liquid on the skin to neutralise the effect of the chemicals in the tape and therefore lessen the risk of skin irritation. I have tried this ever since on all of my patients and it really works. However I never leave a tape on for more than 48 hours and stress that if there is any suggestion of irritation it should be removed immediately.

13. The hip joint.

As with other mobile joints, where possible, the glide with movement should be at right angles to the movement glide. (i.e. Medial or lateral glide with finger flexion).

a. Loss of internal rotation.

One of the movement losses that inculpates the hip joint is internal rotation, and provided the patient does not have too much joint deterioration on X-ray this mobilisation is excellent. Let us assume that your patient has a loss of medial rotation in her right hip.

The MWM can be done in lying or weight bearing.

Lying. The patient lies on a treatment couch with her hip and knee flexed. Your treatment belt is around her upper thigh and around your upper thighs just below your hip joints. It is essential that the belt is as high as it will go on the patient otherwise the belt will be painful and the glide ineffective. Your bent left elbow is now placed in your left groin and the hand is placed on her lateral ilium. The forearm is inside the belt. When in position the belt must have no slack. (See figure 50a). Wrap your right arm around the patient's thigh and lower leg. This is positioned so that you will be able to passively internally rotate the hip while you laterally glide the femur using your thighs to do this via the belt. Your left forearm, positioned as it is, stabilises the pelvis and is the key to the success of the treatment. Using this technique will, in nearly every case, painlessly improve the range of rotation thus improving the patient's function and reducing the pain. Sets of these are done and the patient is encouraged to do appropriate exercises at home.

Standing. With the patient standing, place the belt around his thigh and around your thighs. As you will see from the picture (Figure 50b) the belt lies horizontally. With your hands placed on the patient's ilium, to stabilise it, apply a lateral distraction force using your thighs. Sustain this and have the patient rotate on the affected leg with his other leg held just off the floor. The distraction force need only be applied just short of the limited and/or painful range of rotation. It is ideal if someone can hold the patient's hands while he turns or he has the back or a chair or whatever to grasp for security.

This technique is just as good for external rotation difficulties.

b. To restore hip flexion

The technique set up is exactly the same as for rotation in lying. Instead of passively rotating the hip you passively flex it with your free hand while the glide is applied laterally.

In standing, the patient the patient places his foot on a chair. He holds the back of the chair for security and flexes forward while you apply a sustained lateral distraction with the belt.

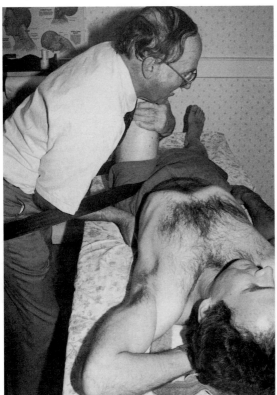

Figure 50a
MWM for hip rotation lying.

Figure 50b
MWM for hip rotation in standing.

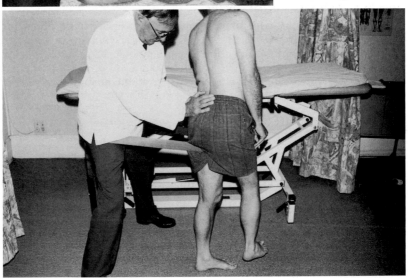

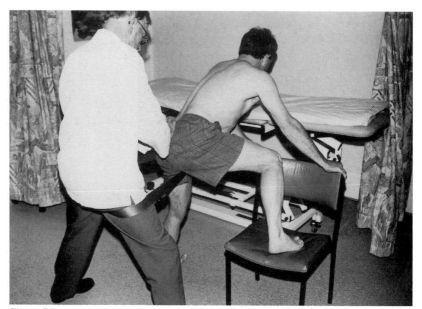

Figure 50c

MWM for hip abduction weightbearing.

c. To restore hip abduction.

The patient stands with his affected leg on the floor and his sound leg's foot on a chair. His legs should be as far apart as possible. He holds the back of the chair for security. When he flexes further his knee on the chair and shifts his pelvis sideways towards it, he will be applying overpressure to the abduction taking place in his troublesome hip. This stretch is accompanied by a posterior glide of his hip joint by you, using a treatment belt. The photo should be self explanatory . (See figure 50c) Your free hands are stabilising his ilium. Try this MWM the next time you have a chronic **adductor strain** to deal with. Things are not always what they seem.

d. To restore hip extension.

The patient stands facing a chair with the foot of his good leg on it. He grasps the back of the chair for security. You stand on the affected side with the belt around his upper thigh as far up as it will go. In the case of males do avoid their "furniture" (This delightful term is used by my accredited teaching colleague Mike Dufresne). Your thighs are also within the belt. You apply a sustained lateral distraction as the patient flexes forward over his knee and then extends his spine. It is like an ilio psoas stretch. (See figure 50d)

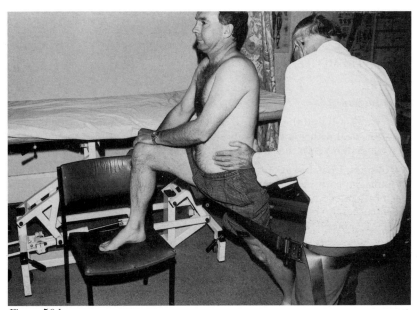

Figure 50d

MWM for hip extension in standing.

14. FINAL COMMENTS ON MOBILISATIONS WITH MOVEMENTS.

Remember with all applications of MWMS for painful joint restrictions, that the direction of your glide is critical. Pain may be produced if you are slightly off the treatment plane. Minor alterations to the gliding direction can make a tremendous difference.

Remember that MWMS when indicated are never painful.

Remember that overpressure is essential to gain the maximum benefit from a MWM.

Remember to do a sufficient number of repetitions as by doing so they have a more lasting effect and seem to restore the options to the joint to stay on track or in position.

Remember to instruct the patients whenever possible to do their own MWMS.

Remember whenever possible to tape the patient's joint in a corrected position for two days and repeat the taping as necessary.

Remember that other forms of therapy can be given concurrently.

Remember to use them as part of your assessment to see if they are indicated.

Finally . . . Remember to use them even if they are revenue reducing.

PART THREE

THE EXTREMITIES. A POT POURRI

Introduction

The reader will find this an unusual title for a treatise on the extremities but I wish to deal with some innovations for old techniques plus some old and new ideas of my own that I am sure physiotherapists will find of value.

In Helsinki, 1970, I went on my first course in manual therapy for the extremity joints. My early mentor Freddy Kaltenborn was the teacher. I have of course been influenced by the teachings of G Maitland whose name is synonymous with manual therapy and many others including J Cyriax, R Elvey, J Mennell and J McConnell. I wish at first to discuss compression as a treatment then write about a new concept that I have been working on which I call the Pain Release Phenomenon ("PRP") to which compression therapy relates. "PRP"s have a wide application. They are still being developed and the reader who understands what I am on about will be able to apply "PRP"s in the treatment of many chronic conditions. These comments should make you wish to read further.

A. COMPRESSION TREATMENTS FOR EXTREMITY JOINTS

Preamble

I started using compressions in treatment regimes soon after reading the excellent article of G D Maitland's "The Hypothesis of Adding Compression When Examining and Treating Synovial Joints" in 1981. Although a very useful tool in manual therapy it soon became apparent that if safe guidelines were not developed and understood then some patients would have their conditions exacerbated and others denied this form of therapy. I would like to elaborate on the guidelines I use and then refer to some specific applications.

1. COMPRESSION AS A TEST

Description

As stated in Maitland's article, when assessing extremity joints you should try a compression test to see if this produces pain. To do this the joint is placed in a biomechanical resting position where all the structures surrounding it are maximally relaxed. You now stabilise the proximal facet with one hand and apply a compressive force on the joint with the other. While maintaining this compression try a series of joint movements to see if they produce pain.

The movements to the joint would be those used in passive testing (e.g. flexion, extension, rotation etc.) or accessory movements (glides).

When using these tests avoid end range movement . You are looking for articular pain and if the joint is moved to end range then the pain experienced may be capsular or ligamentous. Common sense must prevail re the amount of compression used. Excessive force is not needed and if the bone ends are painful it will cause unnecessary distress.

2. COMPRESSION AS A TREATMENT

Description

As already stated compression treatments come under the heading I call the "Pain Release Phenomenon" or conveniently "PRP". I will deal with "PRP"s in detail later in this section but at this point suffice to say that 20 seconds seems to be a "magical" time for compressions as a treatment and other "PRP" treatments. Let me explain further.

If a combination of compression and movement causes pain then repeat the combination for up to 20 seconds to see if the pain disappears. Ensure that the pressure on the articular surfaces remains constant. If the pain increases then STOP immediately. Use no more pressure than that required to just produce the pain. If too much is used then that may be why the pain increases. I cannot over emphasise the importance of using the correct amount of compression. If the pain disappears within 20 seconds then a compression treatment is indicated. This means that you repeat the movement with the same amount of compression. The pain will go again within 20 seconds. Further repetitions see a remarkable change in the response of the joint surfaces. After several repetitions the time for the pain to go drops rapidly. Soon there is virtually no pain with the movement and this should signal the end of the first treatment session. On subsequent visits other movements producing pain with compression would be tried. It may become necessary to apply compression at end range. By this time if the pain goes you know it was still articular. If it does not it would indicate the source of pain is elsewhere. As therapists become skilled in using compressions they will find them more useful than originally thought.

I mentioned that if the pain increased with movement and compression you would stop but if the pain does not abate after 20 seconds can I reiterate that it may be because too much force was used. Try it again with less compression and see what happens.

This 20 second guideline will ensure that no patients are ever exacerbated. The exception to this time span has been the patella. We have found that with some chronic knees 25 seconds would be acceptable. In countries where patients are quick to take action against a therapist if they feel worse these rules will be welcome.

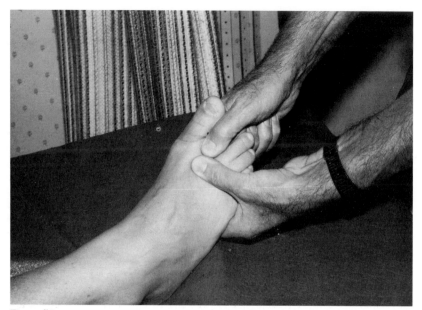

Figure 51

Compression treatment for second metatarso-phalangeal joint.

Some compression applications worth mentioning

N.B. Although I will only mention certain joints remember it is a valid treatment option for any synovial joint where compression pain can be produced.

(1). The metatarso-phalangeal joint of the second toe and perhaps the third or fourth

Patients often present with pain over the heads of their middle metatarsals. It may be diagnosed as metatarsalgia. A compression test is always warranted and if positive then a compression treatment is given. You often get a spectacular result relieving the patient after some months of misery. To do this the patient is lying. You grasp the base of the proximal phalanx of the second toe between your right (or left) thumb and first phalanx of your flexed index finger. The thumb and index finger of your other hand secures the head of the second metatarsal. (See Figure 51) The base of the first phalanx is now glided up and down on the head of the second metatarsal while a moderate compression force is sustained. Try not to pinch when gripping and ensure your glide is a pure one with no wedging. The direction of the glide is oblique and when parallel with the treatment plane the range of movement is unexpectedly considerable when considering the size of the bone ends. If pain is experienced then compress with the glide for up to 20 seconds. If the pain goes within this time span repeat the procedure several times until a satisfactory result is obtained. Remember not to over compress and if the pain increases then stop immediately. As with all the other techniques dealt with in this book other treatments would still be given such as lumbrical exercises etc.

(2). The sesamoids beneath the first metatarso-phalangeal joint

The sesamoids can be suspected of causing weightbearing pain under the base of the big toe when the metatarso- phalangeal joint itself appears on examination to be symptomless.

Compression testing is a valid way of inculpating the wee bones as the cause of pain in their vicinity, under the medial border of the foot. As they are not easy to palpate I use the following routine to test them. Place the lateral border of the fully flexed index finger beneath the sesamoids and opposing thumb on top of the first metatarso-phalangeal joint. Using the flexed index finger provides a larger surface to place under these small bones and ensures they do not escape the compression about to be applied. (See Figure 52). By squeezing with the thumb and index finger so positioned, the sesamoids cannot avoid the compression. You now passively flex and extend the big toe. If pain is produced with this movement then it is probably coming from the sesamoids, particularly if it stops when the compression component is removed. Care must be taken not to compress the tendon of extensor longus hallicus on the

Figure 52

Compression treatment for the sesamoids.

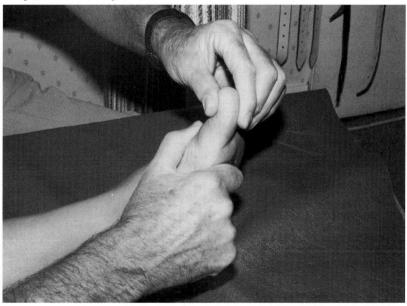

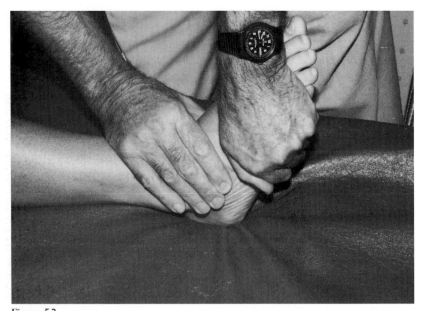

Figure 53

Compression treatment for the metatarso-cuboid joint.

bones beneath as it can be very tender. By off centring the pad of the thumb on top this can be avoided. If compression is painful then use it as a treatment following the 20 second rule. Only a few treatments are usually required. I must mention that I give exercises to strengthen the flexor longus hallicus muscle which is invariably weak and I use 2.5 cm wide zinc oxide strapping to reposition the sesamoids. The latter is done because the sesamoids in the foot are similar to the patella and pathologies can be managed in a similar way. Here I must refer the reader to Jenny McConnell's article "The Management of Chondromalacia Patellar - A Long Term Solution". Her contribution in this field has been immense. The adhesive tape is attached to the sesamoids via the skin which enables them to be pulled medially. To maintain this new position the other end of the tape is wrapped over the dorsum of the foot.

(3). The metatarso-cuboid joint

In my experience I have yet to encounter a restriction between the 4th and 5th metatarsals and the cuboid. However in patients presenting with pain in this joint's vicinity especially on weight bearing a compression test should be given. To do this the patient is lying with his knee on the painful side flexed and his heel on the bed. If the patient's right foot is involved it would be close to the left side of the plinth and you stand at the left side of the patient. You now fixate the cuboid with the right thenar eminence on top and the fingers

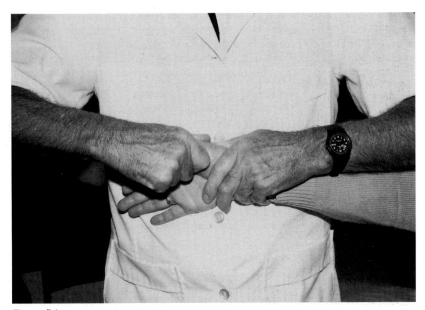

Figure 54

Compression treatment for the trapezium/first metacapal joint.

beneath. The thenar eminence of the other hand together with the fingers grasp the bases and shafts of the 4th and 5th metatarsals. This hand then applies a compression force combined with an antero-posterior glide. (see figure 53). If pain is produced execute a compression treatment regime as discussed in earlier texts.

(4) The trapezium - 1st metacarpal joint

As all physiotherapists know, this is a saddle joint and very prone to degenerative disease. The capsule in the young is slack and it really behaves like a ball and socket joint. If painful the therapist should try a compression test with a view to giving a compression treatment. You hold the seated patient's hand securely to your body. Clasp the trapezium with the thumb and index finger of one hand and the first metacarpal with the thumb and index finger of the other hand (see figure 54). While applying a compressive force, flex and extend then abduct and adduct the thumb to see if it is painful. If so proceed with a compression regime. Provided you follow the 20 second guideline do not be put off by the considerable crepitus sometimes encountered.

(5). The pisiform - triquentrum joint

This joint should not be overlooked when a patient presents with pain in its vicinity. When involved it produces pain with wrist extension especially with passive overpressure as the pisiform is compressed on the carpal beneath. Test this joint by having the patient fully flex the wrist, to relax the structures that stabilise the pisiform, and grasp this small bone with the end pads of the thumb and index finger. It is now compressed on the triquetrum while glided in different directions. If painful apply a compression treatment. I know of no better management.

B. PAIN RELEASE PHENOMENON TECHNIQUES - "PRPS"

Apology

Firstly may I apologise for the use of the initials "PRP" but when writing up case notes etc. they are more convenient. Who wants to keep writing Pain Release Phenomenon Techniques out in full all the time. I am sure you will have a place for them after you have read this section and will choose to use the initials.

1. EXPLANATION AND DESCRIPTION

Physiotherapists have been using techniques that are akin to "PRP"s for many years. When frictions are applied to a lesion we all know that if the pressure is constant and not excessive the tenderness experienced will disappear after a short time. In Part 1 of this book I dealt with the acute wry neck and stated that with repeated rotations into the painful range of movement the pain goes. In the section just covered, I spoke of the pain release phenomenon we look for, within 20 seconds, with compressions. This latter phenomenon led me to try and see if pain would disappear when provoked in other ways and to my astonishment I found that it did. Because of this exciting find, and the correlation with compressions, it had to be covered in this book. As a profession we still have much to learn and do.

At this point in time I would discourage "PRPS" as a therapy for acute conditions. They have a place in the treatment of chronic problems when one can assume that the initial stages of repair have taken place. Let me give an example. Say a patient has just torn some fibres in a muscle. An active contraction would be painful as would a passive stretch. Maintaining the contraction or stretch for 20 seconds would not cause a pain release and the chances are that it would make the lesion worse. This is why I use "PRP"s for conditions of longer standing and 6 weeks as a guideline.

Starting with the lower limb and then the upper limb I will give some applications for "PRP"s .As with other therapies the patient must of course have the purpose of the "PRP"s explained to him. This is because he is expected to feel some discomfort initially and it is important that he informs you as soon as the pain diminishes or goes. When the pain stops it is pointless continuing so they must tell you. You stop and start again. If with your first "PRP" the pain goes in under 6 seconds it may be because you did not provoke enough pain to be useful.

2. SPECIFIC TREATMENT EXAMPLES

(1). *Extensor longus hallucis tendinitis*

"PRP"s have proved helpful in resolving this condition. The diagnosis is confirmed clinically when resisted active toe extension, palpation and a passive stretch of the tendon are all painful. To treat, you give just enough resistance to active big toe extension to produce a tolerable pain in the tendon. The active contraction is maintained for up to 20 seconds to see if the pain goes. An explanation is of course given to the patient of what to expect. I usually get more patient involvement by getting them to monitor the time for me with a watch. If the pain disappears the procedure is repeated several times until the movement is virtually painless. It is interesting to note that with each contraction more resistance is required to produce the same level of pain. The next step would be to produce the pain with a stretch. Follow the 20 second rule and if successful repeat several times. At the time of the first visit it may be advisable to use only one procedure. The patients are taught to do their own "PRP"s. This technique would not be used on an acute tendinitis.

(2). *Hip pain*

Many adults present with hip problems. They may have a capsular pattern loss of movement or have a positive FABER's sign. "PRP"s can make a dramatic change in the patient's symptoms. The patient would be lying supine. Standing on the unaffected side you flex the hip and knee so that the former is at approximately 90 degrees. Adduction is also added. A pad is placed under the patient's buttock on the affected side. One or both of your hands are placed over the flexed knee and a shoulder makes contact with the hand(s) on the knee. (See Figure 55a). By using the body weight through the hand(s) on the knee a dorsal glide is applied to the hip joint. In seeking pain with this glide, variations in flexion and/or adduction may be necessary. You apply the "PRP" routine that will now be coming familiar. It is of course of little use in advanced cases of arthritis and what is more you would not receive a favourable response within the 20 seconds.

The next procedure would be for a patient with a positive FABER's test. Place him in this test position and then press his knee towards the plinth seeking pain at a tolerable level. (See Figure 55b). Maintaining it for the "magical" 20 seconds see if it responds favourably. If so proceed and the knee will move closer to the plinth and the patient will arise feeling much better. You sometimes get fabulous results. Another way to "PRP" is, when in the FABER position, have the patient actively abduct against resistance that you apply. If this produces pain have him hold the contraction for up to 20 seconds and see if the pain subsides. It usually will and subsequent contractions bring the knee closer to the bed. "PRP"s offer much to the therapist and patient in the management of hip pain and stiffness.

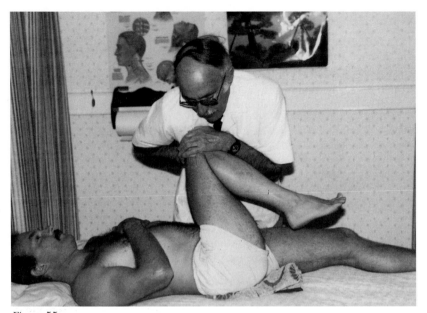

Figure 55a

"PRP" hip joint. Postero-lateral glide of femur.

Figure 55b

"PRP" to hip joint in Faber position.

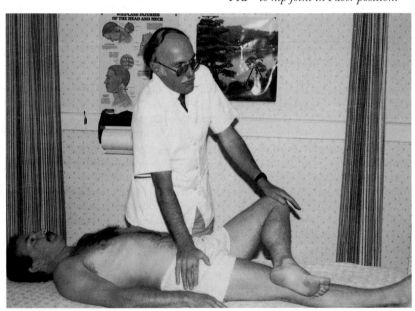

3). De Quervain's disease (stenosing tenovaginitis)

This painful condition is difficult to treat and often requires surgical intervention. However I would suggest you include in your therapy "PRP"s. To do this have the patient make a fist with the thumb inside the fingers. You now deviate the wrist medially until a tolerable level of pain is produced. The patient can in fact do this with the other hand. The "PRP"s are now under way.

(4). Tennis Elbow

With all "PRP"s, as the reader will now be aware, the contractions or stretches which reproduce the pain are sought and from these the treatment strategy is planned. For "tennis elbow" I would suggest that you make use of the tests used in making the diagnosis.

Many patients experience pain with resisted extension of the 4th and/or 3rd fingers. This discomfort is usually worse in full extension of the elbow but you would start at 90 degrees, if this was also pain positive, and use "PRP"s on the painful responses using one finger at a time. The patient is taught to do them and instructed to repeat the program six times a day. Patients responding to this program report pleasing daily progress and it becomes necessary for them to extend the arm further to reproduce the pain. Use is made of other pain provoking movements such as wrist extension with a clenched fist.

However the reader will recall that earlier in this book a new approach in the treatment of tennis elbow was using mobilisations with movement. MWMs should be tried first and if unsuccessful then try the above.

(5). Golfer's Elbow

I first used "PRP"s on a 40 years old patient who, as the result of a direct blow to the medial aspect of his elbow was suffering from a medial epicondylitis. This condition had bothered him for over four months and failed to respond to medication. On examination he was unable to flex his fingers or wrist against any resistance without considerable pain. On the day of his first visit he had ultrasound and then wrist and finger flexion "PRP"s. He was an intelligent patient and was both interested and pleased with his response to this new therapy. He quickly learned to "PRP" himself. Two days later he was virtually pain free and no further treatments were given. This proved to me beyond reasonable doubt that "PRP"s were a valuable adjunct to our therapies.

(6). The chronic painful shoulder

This is indeed a vague heading but I have had some super results using "PRP"s on many of the different conditions that befall the shoulder joint. I seek the static contractions or stretch movements that produce pain and look for the 20 seconds or less response. One procedure that I have found of great value

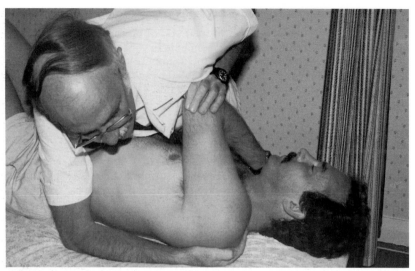

Figure 56

A "PRP" for the shoulder. Similar to hip technique.

has been to have the patient supine on the plinth with his elbow fully flexed and the shoulder flexed to 90 degrees. I am referring to the painful side of course. You stand at the good side and place one hand over the patient's elbow and the other under his scapular. (See Figure 56). Use your body weight to glide the humeral head posteriorly seeking pain. It may be necessary to add some horizontal flexion to the humerus to provoke discomfort. When painful sustain for up to 20 seconds to see if the desired pain disappearance occurs. The procedure is similar to that used on the hip and described earlier. This has proved very useful with some chronic rotator cuff lesions.

3. CONCLUSION

The most exciting thing about "PRP"s is that like other forms of manual therapy the therapist can expect some change at the time of delivery when they are indicated. I laboured this point when dealing with "NAGS" and "SNAGS". However they should not be used to the exclusion of other physical therapies.

The biggest problem that therapists will have with "PRP"s will be judging the amount of resistance to give when applying them or how much stretch to use. It is better to start with too little than too much. If too little the pain produced may only take a few seconds to disappear. One would of course, if this were the case, apply stronger resistance or a stronger stretch the next time. Too much sustained resistance could exacerbate the lesion and "PRP"s might have to be discarded. This "magical" time of 20 seconds may need reconsidering. There have been times with very chronic conditions when I

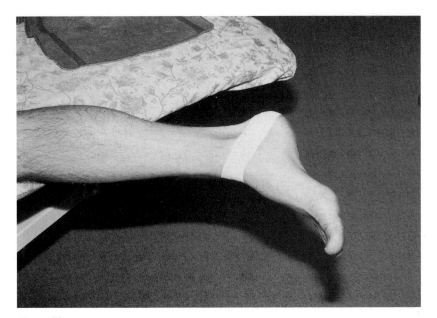

Figure 57
Taping for heel pain.

have lingered longer with good results but there will always be exceptions to rules. I have also mentioned that in the early stages of soft tissue injuries they should not be used but maybe if done gently and looking for say a 5 second pain relief response they may have a place in speeding up recovery. I would hesitate to try them within 48 hours of injury bearing in mind the R.I.C.E. advice. At this point in time my most spectacular results have been with conditions of many months standing.

C. OTHER EXTREMITY THERAPIES

Explanation

In this final section I wish to refer to assorted techniques that the reader will find of interest. This will further explain the use of the term pot pourri in the heading of Part 2. Not to be missed is the "SQUEEZE" technique for the knee.

1. PLANTAR FASCIITIS - HEEL PAIN

In the November 1973 issue of the N.Z. Journal of Physiotherapy I had published an article titled " 'Plantar Fasciitis': A Study Report". This article dealt with heel pain and the inference was that most patients diagnosed as having chronic plantar fasciitis had a joint problem. The sub talar joints were involved and causing the pain and not the plantar fascia. I drew this conclusion from the fact that most patients presenting with heel pain responded to manual therapy to these joints together with exercises and footwear advice.

Years later nothing has happened to make me change my mind and in this respect I have the support of many colleagues.

In this edition I wish to add the strapping that I use for heel pain. It can be so effective that when applied, patients who have limped into my rooms have walked out with no pain. The tape is used to alter the position of the calcaneum in relation to the talus. This is achieved by taping the calcaneum in external rotation. Two strips (approximately 2 cms wide) are used. The first is placed obliquely around the back of the heel, and while the calcaneum is forcibly externally rotated, the tape is wrapped up around the lower leg to maintain the position. The second tape is applied over the first to make the fixation even more effective. (See figure 57) When the patients stand they initially have difficulty walking because of the repositioning but no pain should be felt. The tape is left for 48 hour and the result noted. It is part of the treatment routine for heel pain and may have to be used for three weeks.

2. THE "SQUEEZE" TECHNIQUE FOR THE KNEE

Introduction

The origin of this treatment must be told and before doing so I would again remind the reader of that famous quote attributed to Louis Pasteur ... "In the field of discovery chance only favours the prepared mind". Some years ago we were treating a grubby 25 year old male with a knee joint "derangement". He twisted it playing football resulting in loss of at least 25 degrees of extension and 35 degrees of flexion. Some hours after his injury the knee became swollen and he had a noticeable bulge over the antero - medial joint margin. An appointment had been made for him to see an orthopaedic surgeon and pending this visit he was referred to us for therapy. Our management included the usual manual techniques one may try to restore knee movement, ultrasound and of course quadriceps and hamstring exercises. The therapy was useless and resulted in the patient understandably complaining on his fifth visit that he would be wasting his time by attending further. We readily agreed with him and asked him to maintain an exercise program at home until assessed by the surgeon. As a final gesture I decided to again check his knee. I used the McMurray test and applied a very firm pressure over the anterior horn where the prominent bulge was located. To my amazement while squeezing over the joint margin I was able to flex it fully without pain, and even more amazingly I was then able to extend it fully from the flexed position. It must be added that I did not release my firm thumb pressure over the anterior horn. The patient was understandably delighted. "I'm cured!" he exclaimed. "Of course!" was my nonchalant reply. It was then pointed out to this fellow that only a temporary resolution to his problem had been brought

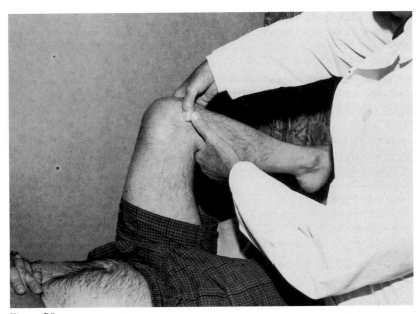

Figure 58a

"Squeeze" technique for the knee. Medial "derangement" in lying.

Figure 58b

"Squeeze" technique in partial weightbearing for medial joint signs.

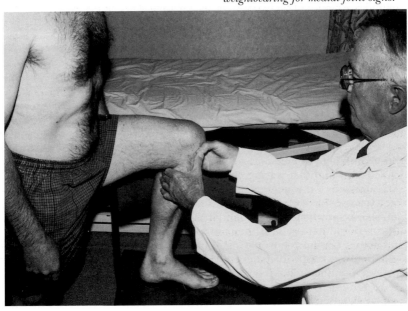

about and he could expect further trouble if he twisted his knee again. He demanded after this "miracle" a return appointment two days later which was agreed to. He was fine and required neither further therapy nor surgery.

Referring again to my quotation above may I say that I most certainly had a prepared mind. From that time the "Squeeze" technique has been an important and rewarding part of my therapy for knees that have lost flexion and in many cases can be helpful in "unlocking" a knee following injury.

The "Squeeze" for flexion can be applied in lying or standing but for extension is only done in lying.

Knee flexion is tested in lying and weightbearing for a movement loss and/ or pain. If the restriction and pain is present when lying then your treatment is done in this position. If the loss and pain is only evident when weightbearing then the "Squeeze" would be applied with the patient standing. Please be mindful of the contraindications to manual therapy and if you have any doubts always give a trial treatment with the patient supine. The treatment is always uncomfortable but not painful and should be well tolerated by the patient.

Before describing the procedure I would draw your attention to the fact that when a knee is put through a full range of movement there is always a position through this range when you can palpably feel some joint space between the femur and tibia. This is because of the very convex shape of the femoral facet and the way the joint behaves biomechanically. In full flexion for instance it is easy to palpate the joint space over the anterior horn of the meniscus (medial or lateral), but with extension this cannot be done as the tibia and femur approximate. One makes use of this knowledge, as the "Squeeze" is applied when you feel there is space available beneath the fingertips during the range of movement.

Description for a loss of flexion

The supine patient's knee is palpated around the medial and lateral joint margins seeking an area of local tenderness. If pain is located over the postero - medial joint space of the right knee you stand at the left side of the patient. Place the medial border of one thumb, reinforced by the other, over the joint margin where it is tender. The patient now actively flexes his knee and when you feel the joint space open up beneath your thumbs you squeeze centrally. At the same time you encourage additional joint flexion with the ulnar border of your hand that is lying over the upper end of the tibia. (See Figure 58a). Maintain the squeeze and overpressure for a few seconds and repeat three times before reassessing the range of movement. Patients will always feel discomfort which is understandable but it is a tolerable procedure and if not you would not use it. If the pain and palpable tenderness was over the lateral joint margin you would stand on the same side to enable you to use your thumbs to apply the squeeze. The thumbs are used because they are stronger than the fingers.

If the pain and/or loss of movement is when weightbearing only then the "Squeeze" is done while the patient squats down. Kneel at your patient's feet and place your thumbs over the joint margin where you suspect attention is needed. As the patient squats you apply thumb pressure as the joint space becomes available. (See Figure 58b). Have the patient hold on to something like the back of a chair for security. This weightbearing variation would also be used as a progression on the supine position if you thought it necessary. Words like exciting should not be used in a textbook to describe what so often happens with this technique. However when you can markedly increase the flexion in a knee that has been absent for 8 years with a "Squeeze" and do this in the presence of many colleagues why not? May I again remind the reader that if the squeeze discomfort increases as a patient bends his knee abandon the technique as you must with other therapies covered in this book. If there is no improvement in range at the time of delivery then try something else.

Explanation

I am always asked when teaching what I think this technique is doing when one considers the known pathologies that occur within the knee. The menisci as we know are wedge shaped. Perhaps a new type of mechanical lesion called "an abnormal meniscal distortion" should be considered. Perhaps with a weightbearing twist of the knee a part of the meniscus can distort slightly in

Figure 59

Fixation of clavicle for acromio-clacicular derangement.

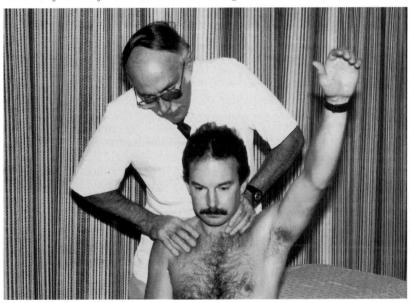

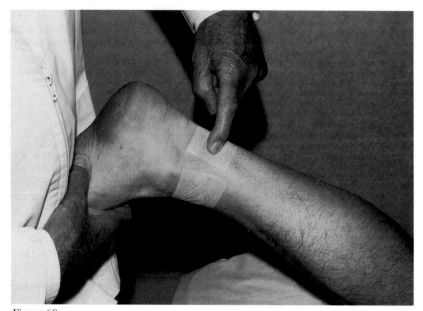

Figure 60

Taping of tendo-achilles for medial tendon pain.

a peripheral direction. It could even do this sometimes when the meniscus is torn. This would explain why squeezing in a remedial direction can spectacularly correct a flexion loss that remains following successful arthroscopic surgical intervention. It works, perhaps you have a better explanation?

3. THE ACROMIO - CLAVICULAR JOINT

According to some anatomists this joint can have a meniscus and I would agree. Often after trauma it responds to a technique I evolved to mobilise the joint and deal with it if deranged. The procedure takes into account the fact that when the arm is fully elevated through flexion the clavicle externally rotates. If this rotation is blocked and the arm elevated actively with some momentum, at the end of the motion an additional rotation will take place at the acromio-clavicular joint. It is the momentum that makes this happen. If you try this on a normal joint you can invariably produce a crepitus. With the injured joint it tends to remain silent if it is hypomobile but after a few swings with clavicular fixation it frees and the patient is instantly much better.

To do this have the patient seated. Stand behind him and to one side and fixate the clavicle on the other side with the ulnar border of your hand. (See Figure 59). The patient now swings his arm up in front of him towards full elevation. He must not be too vigorous. It is important that the therapist does not stand behind the arm being elevated for fear of being struck in the face. However one blow will ensure compliance. I usually have them swing a few times seeking the return of the crepitus. If the patient found it too painful then follow the golden rule and desist.

5. USEFUL TAPINGS (Not already mentioned)

Achilles tendonitis and other soft tissue injuries

For many years we have taped the tendo-achilles laterally when patients present with pain on the medial side of the tendon.(see fig 60) These patients often have pronated feet which, when viewed from behind, makes the tendon convex medially and thus more vulnerable to strain. The taping makes the tendon concave medially and alters the way the foot weightbears. It alters the way the muscle tracks and enables the tendon, when damaged, to recover more rapidly. We would still use modalities etc. Remember to never leave the tape on for more than 48 hours and it must come off immediately if any pain or skin irritation is experienced.

Because this approach has been so successful, we have used the same principle on muscle lesions etc. throughout the body.

With hamstring lesions, if the strain is medial we tape the muscle bulk laterally, if the strain is lateral we tape it medially. The patients trial the tape and remove it if after an hour it does not appear to be helpful. With trochanteric bursitis we tape the tensor fascia lata ventrally or dorsally to alter its tracking over the great trochanter. Very effective.

For acute tennis elbows tape the extensor muscle bulk laterally, to see if it alter the pain with function.

Patients are advised to trial taping and if successful persevere with it. As mentioned before in this text, patients are told to use "MYLANTA" on the skin as it is very helpful in avoiding tape skin reactions.

EPILOGUE

This book was written with one purpose in mind and that was to acquaint the reader with the techniques of the author. The contents could have included copious details of pertinent anatomy and biomechanics but this background material is well known to physiotherapists and there are always many excellent texts available.

My most valuable self learning and teaching tools are my articulated plastic spine and the articulated bones of the upper and lower extremity. Being flexible and accurate in detail makes it simple for me to show and explain to patients what I propose to do. This is especially true for "NAGS", "SNAGS" and "MWMS".

After presenting a paper on "SNAGS" at the 1988 IFOMT World Congress in Cambridge, England I was asked by many participants what the initials NAG stood for. There is of course a tale related to this. For years when recording manual techniques I have related many of them to the source. A Kaltenborn technique was often prefixed with the initials Kb, a Maitland technique would be prefixed with Mait or a McConnell with McC. With my original neck mobilisations I cheekily thought of calling them Nagillums which of course is Mulligan spelt backwards. My colleague of the day, Trish Gardiner, said the word was far too long and shortened it to NAGS. Some years later a bright colleague suggested that NAG could be an acronym for the words Natural Apophyseal Glides which says it all.

Much of what is covered in this book will eventually be supported by sound clinical trials and in fact some already is. I look forward to the future with confidence and enthusiasm. There is still so much to discover and learn which makes life exciting.

INDEX